BOOTHE'S
SMALL ANIMAL FORMULARY SIXTH EDITION

DAWN BOOTHE, DVM, MS, PHD, MS, DIP ACVIM, DIP ACVCP

D15954O4

American Animal Hospital Association Press
12575 West Bayaud Avenue
Lakewood, Colorado 80228
800/252-2242 or 303/986-2800
www.aahanet.org

978-1-58326-097-5

Library of Congress Cataloging-in-Publication Data
Boothe, Dawn Merton.
  Boothe's small animal formulary / Dawn Boothe. – 6th ed.
    p. ; cm.
  ISBN 978-1-58326-097-5 (wire-o-bound : alk. paper) 1. Veterinary prescriptions—Handbooks, manuals, etc. 2. Veterinary drugs—Dosage—Hand-
books, manuals, etc. I. American Animal Hospital Association. II. Title. III. Title: Small animal formulary.
  [DNLM: 1. Drug Therapy—veterinary—Handbooks. 2. Formularies—Handbooks. 3. Veterinary Drugs—administration & dosage—Handbooks. SF
916.5 B725b 2009]

  SF916.5B66 2009
  636.089'5—dc22

                          2008044348

Cover and interior design by Elizabeth Lahey.

CONTENTS

How to Use this Book

This AAHA formulary has evolved significantly since the first edition in 1988. Since 1997, when the fourth edition was published, more than one hundred new drugs have been added. In addition, eight appendices are included for quick reference. An alphabetical list of drugs by generic name and links to their brand names will ensure proper translation when administering or prescribing these drugs to animals. The Classification of Drugs (Generic Name) by Action or Therapeutic Use (Appendix A) that appeared in previous editions has been retained in the current edition. This feature will simplify your search for the ideal drug to use in a specific instance. Each drug is listed by generic name and its corresponding indications, dose, route, and frequency.

The indications listed in the book are intended as a quick guide only. Clinicians should be thoroughly familiar with any drug used in this book and the risks associated with that use. Doses listed are drawn from other publications, which often reflect anecdotal reports. A full presentation of the risks associated with the use of many drugs, including drug interactions, simply is not possible for our purposes. Thus, the information in this book should be used as a guide only. Clinicians are encouraged to discuss with pet owners the risks associated with the use of drugs.

Preface to the Sixth Edition

This version of the AAHA formulary has attempted to maintain attributes from previous editions which make it a user-friendly resource of drug doses while expanding and improving on aspects that have changed in the last eight years since publication of the fifth edition. This includes the addition of new drugs approved for use in dogs and cats. One of the major changes experienced in the last decade is the advent of antimicrobial resistance. As microbes become more resistant to the available drugs, minimum inhibitory concentrations (MIC) change. Antimicrobial dosage regimens should also change; however, information regarding the magnitude of these changes is limited. Accordingly, when using this formulary for the antimicrobial dosing regimens, the user is reminded that regimens should be individualized as much as possible for the patient. This is particularly salient for older antimicrobials where the labeled doses were often promulgated during the approval process, which may have been several decades ago when bacterial susceptibility (MIC) were much lower. To minimize the risk of antimicrobial resistance, doses should be selected such that infecting pathogens are killed. For all drugs, dose increases are also indicated to adjust for tissues that are difficult to penetrate (e.g., sanctuaries in the presence of marked inflammation). For concentration-dependent drugs, dose increases should be considered, and for time-dependent drugs, intervals might be shorted with constant rate infusions (CRI), particularly for those drugs with very short half-lives (e.g., many older beta-lactams). Dosing should ideally be based on pharmacodynamics (e.g., MIC data). It should be noted that the greater the risk that resistance might develop in the patient, the greater the need to adjust doses or intervals to maximize killing concentrations at the site of infections.

The presence of a drug in the formulary does not necessarily indicate that the listed drug is the preferred drug for the indicated use. Additionally, no attempt has been made to indicate level of risk when used at the recommended dose. It is assumed that clinicians have reviewed the risks and benefits associated with the use of any drug listed in the formulary.

Doses of selected drugs, including anticonvulsants and immunomodulators (e.g., cyclosporine), should be based on the combination of therapeutic drug monitoring and clinical response. Many drugs have different dosing regimens. With this edition, an attempt has been made to consolidate differing dosing regimens such that duplication is reduced. The different dosing regimens reflect the long history of anecdotal use that frequently serves as a basis for dosing decisions in veterinary medicine. In this day of evidence-based medicine, a scientific basis for dosing regimens is desirable. Unfortunately, for many doses, this is not a realistic option. For doses that are markedly varied, when a scientific basis could be identified, a preferred dosing regimen was identified and alternatives deleted. When justification for preference could not be identified, all regimens were retained. Sources reviewed for evidence of doses included textbooks,[1-3] refereed or peer-reviewed veterinary scientific journals, package inserts, and alternate drug formularies.[4-7]

The author would like to gratefully acknowledge Harry Boothe, DVM, MS, DACVS, for his editorial attentiveness throughout the preparation of this formulary and Patricia Dowling, DVM, MSc, DACVIM, DACVCP. Dr. Dowling's meticulous review has contributed substantially to the utility of this formulary.

References

1. Boothe DM. *Small Animal Clinical Pharmacology and Therapeutics*. Philadelphia, PA: WB Saunders Co.; 2001.

2. Bonagura, JD, Twedt, DC. *Kirk's Current Veterinary Therapy XIV*. Philadelphia, PA: WB Saunders Co.; 2008.

3. Greene CE. *Infectious Diseases of the Dog and Cat*. 3rd ed. St. Louis, MO: Elsevier; 2006.

4. Plumb DC. *Plumb's Veterinary Drug Handbook*. 6th ed. Stockholm, WI: PharmaVet, Inc.; 2008.

5. Papich MG. *Saunders Handbook of Veterinary Drugs*. 2nd ed. St. Louis, MO: Elsevier; 2007,

6. Allen DG, Dowling PM, Smith DA. *Handbook of Veterinary Drugs*. 3rd ed. Baltimore, MD: Lippincott Williams & Wilkins; 2005.

7. Kuehn DF. *North American Companion Animal FORMULARY*. 8th ed. Port Huron, MI: North American Compendiums, Inc.; 2008.

Drug	Indications	Dose	Route	Frequency (hr)
Acarbose	Hyperglycemia (adjuvant therapy)	25-50 mg (D). Maximum of 100 mg/dog in dogs >25 kg	PO	With each meal
		12.5-20 mg/cat	PO	With each meal
Acemannan	Immunomodulation	2 mg	Intralesional	7 days for a minimum of 6 weeks
		1 mg/kg	IP	7 days
Acepromazine	Preanesthetic	0.025-0.25 mg/kg (D). Maximum of 3 mg	IM, IV, SC	To effect
	Restraint, sedation	0.025-1.13 mg/kg (D). Maximum of 3 mg	IM, IV, SC	To effect
		0.56-2.25 mg/kg (D)	PO	6-8
		0.05-0.1 mg/kg	IV	To effect
		0.05-2.25 mg/kg (C). Maximum of 1 mg	IM, PO, SC	To effect
	Arterial thromboembolism	0.15-0.3 mg/kg	SC	8-12
	Amphetamine toxicosis	0.05-1 mg/kg (10-18 mg/kg if large dose of amphetimine ingested)	IM, IV, SC	To effect

DRUG	INDICATIONS	DOSE	ROUTE	FREQUENCY (HR)
Acetaminophen with codeine	Analgesic	10-15 mg/kg (D) (based on acetaminophen)	PO	8-12
Acetazolamide	Metabolic acidosis	3.3-10 mg/kg (D)	PO	6-8
	Glaucoma	50 mg/kg	IV	Once
		50-75 mg/kg (D)	PO	8-12
		7 mg/kg (C)	PO	8
Acetylcysteine	Respiratory disease	3-6 mL/hr for 30-60 min (D)	Nebulization	12
		125-500 mg	IV, PO	12
	Acetaminophen toxicosis	140 mg/kg	IV	Loading dose
		Loading dose: 140 mg/kg	IV	Once
		Followed by: 70 mg/kg	PO	4-6 x 5-7 treatments
Acetylsalicylic acid	Struvite urolithiasis	12.5 mg/kg (D)	PO	12
Acetylpromazine	See Acepromazine			
Actinomycin D	See Dactinomycin			
Acitretin	Dermatologic	0.5-2 mg/kg (D)	PO	24
	Actinic keratosis	10 mg/cat	PO	24
	Bowen's disease	3 mg/kg (C)	PO	24
Activated charcoal	Gastrointestinal adsorbent	1 g/5-10 mL water. Administer 6-12 mL of slurry/kg; follow with 0.9%	PO	6 h for several days

Drug	Indications	Dose	Route	Frequency (hr)
continued –		saline cathartic		
		1-8 g/kg (granules)	PO	6 h for several days
Acyclovir	Feline herpes	200 mg	PO	6
		10-25 mg/kg	PO	12
Adequan	See Polysulfated glycosoaminoglycans			
Albendazole	*Filaroides hirthi*	25-50 mg/kg (D)	PO	12 x 5 days. Repeat in 21 days
	Filaroides osleri	9.5 mg/kg (D)	PO	12 x 5-10 days
		25 mg/kg (D)	PO	12 x 5 days. Repeat in 14 days
	Capillaria plica	50 mg/kg (D)	PO	12 x 10-14 days
	Paragonimus killicotti	25-50 mg/kg (D)	PO	24 x 14-21 days
		25-50 mg/kg (C)	PO	12-24 x 10-21 days
	Guardia	25 mg/kg	PO	12 x 2-5 days
	Leishmaniosis	10 mg/kg (D)	PO	24 x 30 days
		5 mg/kg (D)	PO	6 x 60 days
	Platynsoum, *Opisthorciidae* (liver flukes)	50 mg/kg	PO	24 until ova are gone
Albuterol	Bronchodilator	0.02-0.05 mg/kg	PO	8-12 x 10 days
		1-3 puffs	Metered dose inhaler	12 to 24

DRUG	INDICATIONS	DOSE	ROUTE	FREQUENCY (HR)
Aldactazide	See Spironolactone/ hydrochlorthiazide			
Alfentanil	Preanesthetic	5 μg/kg	IV	To effect
	Analgesic supplement	2-5 μg/kg	IV	20 min
Allopurinol	Urate urolithiasis	7-10 mg/kg	PO	8-12 x 30 days then q 24
	Dissolution	15 mg/kg	PO	12. In combination with dietary changes
	Leishmaniosis	15 mg/kg	PO	12 x 60 days
Aloe vera cream	Burns	Length of 0.3-0.6 cm (0.125-0.25 inches)	Topical	6 x several days then q 12-24
Alpha-Keri	Skin moisturizer	1 capful to approximately 1-2 liters of water	Topical. Use as a final rinse or spray aerosol on to wet coat and rub well	6 x several days then q 12-24
Alprazolam	Behavioral problems	0.125-0.25 mg/cat	PO	8-24
		0.01-0.1 mg/kg. Maximum of 4 mg/day	PO	PRN
	Behavioral problems	0.22-0.4 mg/kg	PO	4
		0.25-2 mg/dog	PO	6-12

4

DRUG	INDICATIONS	DOSE	ROUTE	FREQUENCY (HR)
Altrenogest	Luteal deficiency	0.097 mg/kg	PO	24
Aluminum carbonate gel	Phosphate binder	10-30 mg/kg	PO (with food)	8
Aluminum hydroxide	Antacid	2-30 mL	PO	2-4
	Phosphate binder	30-90 mg/kg	PO (with food)	8-24
Aluminum magnesium hydroxide	Laxative	2-10 mL	PO	2-4
Amantadine	Combination analgesia	1.25-4 mg/kg (D)	PO	12-24
		3 mg/kg (C)	PO	24
Amikacin	*Susceptible bacterial infections	15-22 mg/kg	IM, IV, SC	24; consider monitoring (See Appendix F)
Aminocaproic acid (EACA)	Degenerative myelopathy	500 mg/dog	PO	8
Aminopentamide	Antidiarrheal	0.1-0.4 mg	IM, PO, SC	8-12
		0.01-0.03 mg/kg	IM, PO, SC	8-12
		0.1 mg/cat	IM, PO, SC	8-12

DRUG	INDICATIONS	DOSE	ROUTE	FREQUENCY (HR)
Aminophylline (approximately 80% Theophylline)	Bronchodilator	5-11 mg/kg (D)	IM, IV, PO	8-12
		4-6.6 mg/kg (C)	PO	8-12
		2-5 mg/kg (C)	IV (slow)	12
Aminopromazine	Smooth muscle relaxant	2-4.5 mg/kg	IM (D), IV (D), PO(C)	12
6-aminosalicylic acid	See Mesalamine			
Amiodarone	Antiarrhythmic	Initial dose: 10-25 mg/kg	PO	12 x 7 days
		Followed by: 5-7.5 mg/kg	PO	12 x 14 days
		Thereafter: 7.5 mg/kg	PO	24
	Doberman cardiomyopathy	Initial dose: 10 mg/kg	PO	12 x 7 days
		Thereafter: 8 mg/kg	PO	24
Amitraz	Demodectic and sarcoptic mange	19.6 mg/mL	Dip wet dog then air-dry	7-14 days x 3-6 treatments
	Ear mites	Mix 19.6 mg amitraz in 10-20 mL mineral oil	Topical	48 x 3 weeks
Amitriptyline	Behavioral problems, pruritis, neuropathic pain	1-4.4 mg/kg (D)	PO	12-24. Taper withdrawl
	Behavioral problems, urine	5-12.5 mg/cat	PO	24. Taper withdrawl

DRUG	INDICATIONS	DOSE	ROUTE	FREQUENCY (HR)
continued—	spraying, feline lower urinary tract disease			
		1-2 mg/kg (C)	PO	12. Taper withdrawl
Amlodipine besylate	Systemic hypertension	0.625 mg/cat. Increase to 1.25 mg/cat if needed	PO	24
		0.125-0.25 mg/kg (C)	PO	24
		0.1 mg/kg (D)	PO	12 initially then slowly increase (weekly) to
		0.2-0.4 mg/kg (D)	PO	24
Ammonium chloride	Urinary acidifier or struvite dissolution	65 mg/kg (D)	PO	6-12
		800 mg/cat (approximately 1.2 mL, 0.25 tsp, or 1.5% of diet)	PO (with food)	24
		20 mg/kg	PO	8 (D) 12 (C)
	Ammonium tolerance test	0.1 mg/kg of 5% solution	Per rectum	Once
		100 mg/kg. Maximum of 3 g	PO	Once
Amoxicillin	*Susceptible bacterial infections	20-30 mg/kg	IM, IV, PO, SC	6-12
Amoxicillin/clavulanic	*Susceptible bacterial infections	10-30 mg/kg	PO	6-12

Drug	Indications	Dose	Route	Frequency (hr)
continued–		12.5-25 mg/kg (D)	PO	6-12
		62.5 mg/cat	PO	6-12
Amphetamine SO₄	CNS stimulation during certain toxicoses; chlorpromazine overdose	0.5-4 mg/kg (D)	SC	PRN
		5 mg/cat	PO	24 x 4 days
Amphotericin B	Test dose	0.25-0.5 mg/kg	IV	Once
	General mycoses	0.15-1 mg/kg in 30 mL 5% D/W	Rapid IV infusion (over 5 min through a butterfly catheter after flushing catheter with 10 mL 5% dextrose)	48 or 3 x per week to a cumulative dose of 4-12 mg/kg (D) or 4-6 mg/kg (C)
		0.15-1 mg/kg in 200-500 mL 5% D/W via peripheral venous catheter. Dilution of the total dose in 250-400 ml fluid administered SC has been described for cats	IV (over 4-6 hrs)	48 or 3 x per week to a cumulative dose of 4-12 mg/kg (D) or 4-6 mg/kg (C)
	Blastomycosis	Initial dose: 0.5 mg/kg (D)	IV	3 x per week to a cummulative dose of 4-6 mg with ketaconazole
		Followed by: 0.15-0.25 mg/kg (D)	IV	1 x per month with ketaconazole
	Cryptococcosis	0.5-0.8 mg/kg	SC	2-3 x per week. Dilute to <20 mg/mL in 5% dextrose
		0.15-0.4 mg/kg (C)	IV	2-3 x per week for 3-4 weeks.

DRUG	INDICATIONS	DOSE	ROUTE	FREQUENCY (HR)
continued—				Total cumulative dose of 4-6 mg/kg with flucytosine
	Histoplasmosis	Initial dose: 0.5 mg/kg (D)	IV	3 x per week to a cummulative dose of 4-6 mg/kg with ketaconazole
		Followed by: 0.15-0.25 mg/kg	IV	1 x per month with ketaconazole
		0.25 mg/kg (C)	IV	48 x 4-8 weeks with ketaconazole
		0.15-0.5 mg/kg (C)	IV	1 x per month with ketaconazole
	Gastroinestinal pythiosis	1-2 mg/kg (D)	IV	3 x per week to a cumulative dose of 12-24 mg/kg
	Resistant filamentous fungi	2-2.5 mg/kg	IV	3 x per week to a cumulative dose of 15-30 mg/kg
	Leishmaniosis	0.5-0.8 mg/kg	IV	48 to a cumulative dose of 8-16 mg/kg
	Pulmonary fungal disease	Systemic dose diluted in 5% D/W	Aerosol (nebulization)	Use the chosen systemic dose, prepared as 5 mg/mL in 5% dextrose
	CNS fungal disease	0.2-0.5 mg	Intrathecal	2-3 x per week. Dilute in 5 mL cerebral spinal fluid or 10% dextrose
	Fungal cystitis	50 μg/mL prepared in 5% D/W	Urinary bladder infusion	24. Repeat once if necessary

Drug	Indications	Dose	Route	Frequency (hr)
Amphotericin B, colloidal dispersion	Test dose	0.25-0.5 mg/kg	IV	Once
	General mycoses	1-2.5 mg/kg	IV	3 x per week to a cumulative dose of 15-30 mg/kg
Amphotericin B, lipid complex solution	Test dose	0.25-0.5 mg/kg	IV	Once
	General mycoses	1-2.5 mg/kg	IV	3 x per week to a cumulative dose of 15-30 mg/kg
	Blastomycosis, severe	1-2 mg/kg (D)	IV	3 x per week to a cummulative dose of 12-24 mg/kg
	Cryptococcosis	1 mg/kg (C)	IV	3 x per week to cumulative dose of 12 mg/kg
Amphotericin B, liposomal	Test dose	0.25-0.5 mg/kg	IV	Once
	General mycoses	3-4 mg/kg (D)	IV	3 x per week to a cumulative dose of 15-30 mg/kg
	Leishmaniosis	3-4 mg/kg (D)	IV	3 x per week to a cumulative dose of 15-30 mg/kg
Ampicillin	*Susceptible bacterial infections	20-60 mg/kg	PO	6-8
		10-50 mg/kg	IV	6-8

11

Drug	Indications	Dose	Route	Frequency (hr)
Ampicillin sulbactam	*Susceptible bacterial infections	10-50 mg/kg	IM, IV	6-8
Ampicillin trihydrate	*Susceptible bacterial infections	10-50 mg/kg	IM, SC	6-8
Amprolium	Coccidiosis treatment	100 mg/dog	PO (on food or in water)	24 x 7-10 days
		250-300 mg/(D)	PO (on food)	24 x 7-12 days
		60-100 mg (C)	PO	24 x 5 days
		300-400 mg (C)	PO (on food)	24 x 5 days
	Coccidiosis prophylaxis	28.8 mg/L water	PO (in water)	24 x 14 days
		1.25 g of 20% powder	PO (on food)	24 x 14 days
	Coccidiosis treatment	150 mg/kg	PO	24 x 14 days with sulfadimethoxine
Amrinone	See Inamrinone			
Antazoline 0.5%	Allergic conjunctivitis	See label instructions	Topical	24
Antimony	Leishmaniosis	10-50 mg/kg (D)	IV	24 x 10 days. Wait 10 days then repeat
Antivenin	Snake bite	1-5 vials (10-50 mL) (D)	IV	2, PRN
		1-2 vials (D)	IV	4-6, PRN

DRUG	INDICATION	DOSE	ROUTE	FREQUENCY (HR)
Apomorphine	Emesis	0.02-0.04 mg/kg (D)	IM, IV	Efficacy lost with subsequent doses
		0.08-0.1 mg/kg (D)	IM, SC	Efficacy lost with subsequent doses
		0.25 mg	Topical (conjunctival sac)	Flush once emesis begins; efficacy lost with subsequent doses
Aprindine	Ventricular arrhythmias	1-2 mg/kg (D). Maximum of 100 mg	PO	12
		0.1 mg/kg/min (D)	IV (over 5 min)	To effect
Aprotinin	Pancreatitis (protease inhibitor)	5,000 kallikrein inhibitor units (KIU)/kg	IP (preferred), IV	6-8
Ascorbic acid	Copper-induced hepatotoxicity	500-1,000 mg/day (D)	PO	24
	Feline infections peritonitis	25 mg/kg or 125 mg (C)	PO	24
	Acetaminophen toxicosis	30 mg/kg (C)	PO, SC	6 x 7 treatments
	Urinary acidifier	100-500 mg (D)	PO	8-24
		100 mg (C)	PO	8-24
Asparaginase	Lymphosarcoma	10,000 Units/m^2 (small D, C)	IP, IM, IV, SC	7 days as part of a protocol
		30,000 Units/m^2 (large D)	IP, IM, IV, SC	7 days as part of a protocol
	Immune thrombocytopenia	400 Units/kg (D)	IP, IM, IV, SC	Once

DRUG	INDICATIONS	DOSE	ROUTE	FREQUENCY (HR)
continued—	Sterile pyogranulomas	10,000 Units/dog	IP, IM, IV, SC	Once weekly x 1-3 treatments
	Neoplastic disease	10,000 Units/m² (C)	IP, IM, IV, SC	Once weekly x 1-3 treatments
	Combination protocol for neoplasia	400 Units/kg (C)	SC, IM	As protocol indicates
Aspirin	Antipyretic	10 mg/kg (D)	PO	12. For monitoring, (See Appendix F)
		6-10 mg/kg (C)	PO	48-72
	Antithrombotic therapy	5-10 mg/kg (D)	PO	12-48
		6-25 mg/kg (C)	PO	2 x per week
		80 mg/cat	PO	48
	Musculoskeletal pain	25-35 mg/kg (D)	PO	8
	Analgesia, general	10 mg/kg (C)	PO	48
	Antiinflammatory	10-25 mg/kg (D)	PO	8-12
		10-20 mg/kg (C)	PO	48
	Antirheumatic	40-80 mg/cat	PO	48-72
		50 mg/kg (D)	PO	8-12
	Hypertrophic cardiomyopathy	160 mg/cat	PO	2 x per week
	Postadulticide heartworm	5-10 mg/kg (D)	PO	24
	Disseminated Intravascular Coagulation	7.5-15 mg/kg	PO	24-48 x 10 days. Use lower dose if other anticoagulants are concurrently administered

DRUG	INDICATIONS	DOSE	ROUTE	FREQUENCY (HR)
Astemizole	Antihistamine (allergies)	0.2-1 mg/kg (D)	PO	24
Atenolol	Beta blockade	6.25-50 mg (D)	PO	12
		0.25-1 mg/kg (D)	PO	12-24
		2-3 mg/kg (C)	PO	12-24
		5-12.5 mg/cat	PO	24
	Hypertension	2 mg/kg	PO	24
Atipamazole	Reversal agent for medetomidine	Volume equivalent to medetomidine	IV	PRN
Atovaquaone	Antiprotozoal (pneumocystosis)	13.3 mg/kg	PO (with a fatty meal)	8 x 21 days
Atracurium besylate	Paralytic agent	0.2 mg/kg	IV	Initial dose
		0.11 mg/kg	IV	Intraoperative
		4-9 μg/kg/min	CRI	(See Appendix H)
Atropine	Sinus bradycardia	0.022-0.044 mg/kg	IM, IV, SC	To effect
		0.04 mg/kg	PO	6-8
	Atropine response test	0.044 mg/kg	IV	Once
	Preanesthetic	0.02-0.045 mg/kg	IM, IV, SC	PRN
	Hypersialism	0.02 mg/kg	SC	PRN
	Cholinergic toxins	0.2-2 mg/kg	Administer 0.25 the	To effect

Drug	Indications	Dose	Route	Frequency (hr)
continued—			total dose IV and the remaining dose SC, IM	
Auranofin	Autoimmune skin diseases	0.05-0.2 mg/kg (D). Maximum of 9 mg/day	PO	12
Aurothioglucose	Pemphigus complex, plasmacytic stomatitis, and pododermatitis	1st week: 5-10 mg/dog or 1 mg/small dog or cat	IM	Once
		2nd week: 10 mg/dog or 2 mg/small dog or cat	IM	Once
		Then: 1 mg/kg (D, C)	IM	7 days then decrease to once monthly with response
Azathioprine	Immunosuppression, general	2-2.5 mg/kg (D)	PO	24-48
		50 mg/m^2 (D)	PO	24-48
		0.2-1.1 mg/kg (C)	PO	48
	Immune hemolytic anemia	2 mg/kg (D)	PO	24 x 7 days then q 48
	Immune thrombocytopenia	2 mg/kg	PO	24 to effect then taper to
		0.5-1 mg/kg	PO	48
	Myasthenia gravis	2 mg/kg (D)	PO	24 x 7 days then q 48
	Chronic atrophic gastritis	0.5 mg/kg (D)	PO	24-48

DRUG	INDICATIONS	DOSE	ROUTE	FREQUENCY (HR)
continued—	Lymphocytic or eosinophilic enteritis	2-2.5 mg/kg (D)	PO	24-48
		0.2-0.3 mg/kg (C)	PO	24-48
	Chronic active hepatitis	2-2.5 mg/kg (D)	PO	24
	Systemic lupus erythematosus	2.2 mg/kg or 50 mg/m^2 (D)	PO	24-48
	Rheumatoid arthritis	2 mg/kg	PO	24 x 14-21 days then q 48
	Blepharitis, episcleritis	2 mg/kg (D)	PO	24
	Immune polymyositis, masticatory myositis	2 mg/kg	PO	24
Azrithromycin	*Susceptible bacterial infections	5-10 mg/kg (D)	PO	12-24
		3.3 mg/kg (D)	PO	24
		10 mg/kg (D)	PO	5 days
	*Susceptible bacterial infections	7-15 mg/kg (C)	PO	12-24
		5 mg/kg (C)	PO	24-48
Aztreonam	*Susceptible bacterial infections	12-25 mg/kg	IM, IV	8-12
Baclofen	Functional urethral obstruction	5-10 mg/dog	PO	8
		1-2 mg/kg (D)	PO	8
BAL	See Dimercaprol			

16

Drug	Indications	Dose	Route	Frequency (hr)
Baquiloprim/sulfamethoxine or sulphadimidine	Coccidiosis	30 mg/kg	PO	48 x 2 treatments
	*Susceptible bacterial infections	30 mg/kg	PO	24 x 2 days then q 48 x 10-21 days
Beclomethasone diproprionate	Antiinflammatory	200 mg/cat	Metered dose inhaler	PRN
Benazepril	Afterload reduction or hypertension	0.25-1 mg/kg	PO	24
	Renal disease	0.5-1 mg/kg (C)	PO	24
		0.25-0.5 mg/kg (D)	PO	24
Benzimidazole	Trypanosomiosis	5 mg/kg	PO	24 x 2 months
Benzocaine	Local anesthetic	Local	Topical	PRN
Benzoyl peroxide	Seborrheic, antibacterial	Topical	Topical. Leave on skin for 10 min then rinse	Every 3-4 days then decrease to 1 x every 1-2 weeks
Betamethasone	Pannus, episcleritis	1-2 mg/dog	Topical (subconjunctivally)	Decreasing dose: q 5 x 5 days, q 6 x 4 days, q 8 x 3 days, q 12

DRUG	INDICATIONS	DOSE	ROUTE	FREQUENCY (HR)
continued—				x 2 days, then q 24 x 1 day
		0.15 mg/kg (D)	IM	Once
		0.1-0.2 mg/kg	PO	12-24
Bethanechol	Urinary bladder atony, dysautonomia	2.5-25 mg/dog	PO	8
		5-10 mg/dog	SC	8
		1.25-7.5 mg/cat	PO	8-12
Bisacodyl	Stool softener	5-20 mg/dog	PO	24 or PRN
		2-5 mg/cat	PO	24 or PRN
		1-3 suppositories	Per rectum	24 or PRN
		1-2 mL enema	Per rectum	24 or PRN
Bismuth subsalicylate	Gastrointestinal tract protectant	175-524 mg/dog	PO	4-6
		4.4-52 mg/kg (D)	PO	6-8
		4.4 mg/kg (C)	PO	4-6
		18-52 mg/cat	PO	4-6
Bismuth subcarbonate	Gastrointestinal tract protectant	0.3-3 g	PO	4
Bitolerol	Bronchodilation	1-3 puffs	Metered dose inhaler	12 to 24

DRUG	INDICATIONS	DOSE	ROUTE	FREQUENCY (HR)
Bleomycin	Anticancer	$10\ \mu g/m^2$. Maximum dose of $200\ mg/m^2$	IV, SC	24 x 4 days then q 7 days
		0.3-0.5 mg/kg	IM, IV (over 10 min), 1 x per week SC	
Bran	Bulk laxative	Approximately 15-30 mL (1-2 tbsp)/ 400 g food	PO	PRN
Bretylium tosylate	Refractory ventricular arrhythmias	5-10 mg over 8 min	1-2 mg/min	q 1-2 PRN to control arrythmias
Brewer's yeast	Source of B vitamins	0.2 g/kg	PO	24-96
Bromide, potassium or sodium	Anticonvulsant	Loading dose: 90-150 mg/kg	PO (with food)	5 days for a total of 450-600 mg/kg
		Maintenance: 30-90 mg/kg	PO (with food)	24; monitor (See Appendix F)
Bromocriptine mesylate	Hyperadrenocorticism, pseudo-pregnancy	10-30 $\mu g/kg$	PO	24 x 10-16 days
		10-100 $\mu g/kg$	PO	12 x 10-14 days
	Abortifacient	50-100 $\mu g/kg$	IM, PO	24 x 4-7 days 35-45 days after leutenizing hormone surge

Drug	Indications	Dose	Route	Frequency (hr)
Budesonide	Inflammatory bowel disease	1 mg/small dog or cat	PO	24
		2 mg/large dog	PO	24
Bunamidine	Tapeworms (taenia and dipylidium)	20-50 mg/kg	PO	Once after a 3 hour fast
Bupivacaine hydrochloride	Epidural analgesia	0.22-0.3 mL of 0.5% (max 6 mL/dog) (preservative free, methylparaben okay)	Epidural	Once
	Local anesthetic	0.5-1 mL of 0.25% solution	Topical, local	Once
		0.22 mL/kg	Intraarticular	Once
		1.5 mg/kg in 10 to 15 ml saline	Intrathoracic, intraabdominal	Once
Buprenorphine	Analgesia	<11 kg: 15 μg/kg (D)	IM, IV, SC	4-8
		11-23 kg: 10 μg/kg (D)	IM, IV, SC	4-8
		>23 kg: 5 μg/kg (D)	IM, IV, SC	4-8
		5-30 μg/kg (D)	IM, IV, SC, epidural	4-8
		5-30 μg/kg (C)	IM, IV, SC, topical (buccal)	12
Buspirone	Behavioral disorders, anxiolytic	2.5-15 mg/dog	PO	12-8
		1 mg/kg (D)	PO	8-24

Drug	Indications	Dose	Route	Frequency (hr)
continued—		2.5-5 mg/cat	PO	12
		0.5-1 mg/kg (C)	PO	8-12
Busulfan	Chronic myelocytic leukemia	3-4 mg/m²	PO	24
		0.1 mg/kg	PO	24
Butamisole	Hookworms, whipworms	2.2 mg/kg (0.22 mL/kg)	SC	Once then repeat in 21 days
Butorphanol	Antitussive	0.05-0.12 mg/kg (D)	PO, SC	8-12
		0.55-1.1 mg/kg (D)	PO	6-12
	Preanesthetic	0.05-0.4 mg/kg	IM, IV, SC	To effect. (See Appendix H)
	Analgesia, sedation	0.1-1 mg/kg	IM, IV, SC	1-6
		0.55-1.1 mg/kg	PO	6-12
	Antiemetic	0.2-0.6 mg/kg	IM, SC	Once prior to chemotherapy
Cabergoline	Inducing or synchronizing estrus	5 µg/kg	PO	24 x 4-25 days
	Pseudopregnancy	5 µg/kg	SC	24 x 5-10 days
	Abortifacient	5 µg/kg	PO	24 x 7-13 days, 30 days postcoitus in combination with cloprestenol
		5-15 µg/kg	PO	24 x 5 days
		1.7 µg/kg	SC	24 x 6 days

BC

Drug	Indications	Dose	Route	Frequency (hr)
Calcitonin	Hypercalcemia, cholecalciferol toxicosis	Loading dose: 4-6 IU/kg (D)	IV	Once
		Maintenance dose: 4-7 IU/kg (D)	IV, SC	8-12
Calcitriol (Vitamin D$_3$)	Hypoparathyroidism	2.5-3 ng/kg	PO	24
Calcium acetate (contains 23.5% elemental calcium)	Nutritional supplement	2.5 mL (0.5 tsp)	PO	With each meal
	Hypocalcemia	50-75 mg/kg (D)	PO	Divide dose and administer q 8-12
	Phosphate binder	60-100 mg/kg	PO	24
Calcium carbonate (contains 40% elemental calcium)	Hypocalcemia	20-100 mg/kg (D)	PO	8
	Antacid	0.5-5 g/dog	PO	PRN
Calcium chloride (contains 27% elemental calcium)	Ventricular asystole	0.1-0.3 mL/kg of a 10% solution (100 mg/mL)	IV (slowly)	To effect
	Hypocalcemia	0.068-0.13 mEq/kg (0.05-0.1 mL/kg of a 10% solution)	IV (slowly)	To effect

DRUG	INDICATIONS	DOSE	ROUTE	FREQUENCY (HR)
Calcium citrate (contains 21% elemental calcium)	Calcium supplement	10-30 mg/kg	PO (with food)	8
	Urothiliasis	10-30 mg/kg	PO (with food)	8
Calcium EDTA	See Edetate calcium disodium			
Calcium gluconate (contains 9% elemental calcium	Ventricular asystole	0.5-1.5 mL/kg of a 10% solution (100 mg/ml)	IV (slowly)	To effect
Calcium acetate (contains 23.5% elemental calcium)	Hypocalcemia, hyperkalemia	0.225-0.675 mEq/kg (0.5-1.5 ml/kg of 10% solution) (100 mg/ml)	IV (slowly over 20-30 min)	6-8
		25-140 mg/kg	IV (slowly over 20-30 min)	6-8
		50-150 mg/kg 10-15 mg/kg/hr (D)	IV infusion CRI	24 (See Appendix H)
		150-250 mg/kg	PO	8-12
Calcium glubionate (contains 9% elemental calcium)	Hypocalcemia	0.8-1.6 mL/kg (0.165-0.33 tsp) to deliver 25-50 mg/kg elemental calcium	PO	24
Calcium lactate	Hypocalcemia	0.5-2 g/dog	PO	8-24

DRUG	INDICATIONS	DOSE	ROUTE	FREQUENCY (HR)
continued—(contains 13% elemental calcium)		130-200 mg/kg (D)	PO	8
		0.2-0.5 g	PO	24
Captan powder 50%	Dermatomycoses	30 mL/1 L of water (2 tbsp/gal of water)	Topical. Do not rinse	2-3 x per week
Captopril	Vasodilator	0.25-2 mg/kg (D)	PO	8-12
	Congestive heart failure	2-3 mg/cat	PO	8
		3-6.25 mg/cat	PO	12
	Hypertension	0.5-2.0 mg/kg (D)	PO	8-12
Carbamazepine	Anticonvulsant	15-20 mg/dog	PO	12
		2-3 mg/kg (D)	PO	8-12
Carbegoline	Mismating	5 μg/kg (with closprostenol)	PO	24 x 5
Carbenicillin	*Susceptible bacterial infections	15-110 mg/kg	IM, IV, SC	6-8
Carbenicillin indanyl sodium	Urinary tract infections	10-55 mg/kg	PO	8

DRUG	INDICATIONS	DOSE	ROUTE	FREQUENCY (HR)
Carbimazole	Hyperthyroidism	Induction: 5 mg/cat	PO	8 until response then maintenance
		Maintenance: 5 mg/cat	PO	12
Carboplatin	Anticancer	300 mg/m² (D)	IV	Once q 3-4 weeks
		180-260 mg/m² (C)	IV	Once q 3-4 weeks
	Squamous cell carcinoma	100 mg/m² (C)	Intralesional (nasal)	Once q 3-4 weeks
		1.5 mg prepared in purified sesame oil/cm³	Intralesional	7 days x 4 weeks
Carmustine	Anticancer	50 mg/m²	IV	Once q 6 weeks
L-Carnitine	Nutritional supplement, cardio-myopathy	2 g/dog	PO	8-12
		220 mg/kg (D)	IV, PO	24
		250-500 mg (C)	PO	24 x 2-4 weeks
Carprofen	Antiinflammatory, osteoarthritis	4.4 mg/kg (D)	PO, SC	24 or divide dose and administer q 12
	Musculoskeletal pain	4.4 mg/kg (D)	PO, SC	24 or divide dose and administer q 12
	Perioperative pain	2.2-4.4 mg/kg (D)	PO, SC	2 hours prior to surgery
	Postoperative pain	4.4 mg/kg (D)	PO, SC	24 or divide dose and administer q 12
		4 mg/kg (C)	SC	Once
Carvedilol	Cardiac beta blockade	0.5-0.9 mg/kg	PO	12 to effect

DRUG	INDICATIONS	DOSE	ROUTE	FREQUENCY (HR)
Cascara sagrada	Laxative, stool softener	1-4 mL/dog	PO	12 to effect
		0.5-1.5 mL/cat	PO	12 to effect
Castor oil	Cathartic, stool softener	8-30 mL/dog	PO	12 to effect
		4-10 mL/cat	PO	12 to effect
Cefaclor	*Susceptible bacterial infections 4-20 mg/kg		PO (in a fasted animal)	8
Cefadroxil	*Susceptible bacterial infections 20-35 mg/kg		PO	8-12
Cefamandole	*Susceptible bacterial infections 6-40 mg/kg		IM, IV	6-8
Cefazolin sodium	*Susceptible bacterial infections 10-25 mg/kg		IM, IV, SC	6-8
	Acute abdomen syndrome	10-25 mg/kg	IM, IV	4-8
	Surgical prophylaxis	10-22 mg/kg	IV	1-2 times during surgery
Cefepime	*Susceptible bacterial infections 50 mg/kg		IM, IV	8
Cefixime hydrochloride	*Susceptible bacterial infections 5-12.5 mg/kg		PO	12-24
Cefmetazole sodium	*Susceptible bacterial infections 20 mg/kg		IV	6-12
	Surgical prophylaxis	20 mg/kg	IV	Once
Cefoperazone sodium	*Susceptible bacterial infections 22 mg/kg		IV, IM	6-12
Cefotaxime sodium	Acute pancreatitis, osteomyelitis	20-80 mg/kg (D)	IM, IV, SC	4-12
		20-80 mg/kg (C)	IM, IV	8
Cefotetan disodium	*Susceptible bacterial infections 30 mg/kg		IV, SC	8

Drug	Indications	Dose	Route	Frequency (hr)
Cefovecin	*Susceptible bacterial infections	8 mg/kg	SC	7-14 days. More frequent adminstration may be indicated for organisms with higher minimum inhibition concentration (MIC)
Cefoxitin sodium	*Susceptible bacterial infections	15-30 mg/kg (D)	IM, IV, SC	6-8
		6-40 mg/kg (D)	IV	6-8
		11-30 mg/kg (C)	IM, IV	8
	Meningitis, perioperative	20-40 mg/kg (D)	IV	8
Cefpodoxime proxetil	*Susceptible bacterial infections	5-10 mg/kg	PO	12-24
Ceftazidime	*Susceptible bacterial infections		15-30 mg/kg	IM, IV, SC 6-12
Ceftiofur	*Susceptible urinary tract infections	2.2-4.4 mg/kg	SC	12-24
Ceftizoxime	*Susceptible bacterial infections	25-50 mg/kg	IM, IV	8-12
Ceftriaxone	*Susceptible bacterial infections	15-50 mg/kg	IM, IV	12
	Surgical prophylaxis	25 mg/kg	IM, IV	Once
Cefuroxime axetil or sodium	*Susceptible bacterial infections	10-30 mg/kg	IV, PO (with food)	8-12
Cephalexin	*Susceptible bacterial infections	20-60 mg/kg	PO	6-12

DRUG	INDICATIONS	DOSE	ROUTE	FREQUENCY (HR)
Cephalothin	*Susceptible bacterial infections	10-44 mg/kg	IM, IV, SC	4-8
Cephamandole	*Susceptible bacterial infections	6-40 mg/kg	IM, IV	6-8
Cephapirin	*Susceptible bacterial infections	10-30 mg/kg	IM, IV, SC	4-8
Cephradine	*Susceptible bacterial infections	10-40 mg/kg	IM, IV, PO	6-8
Cetacaine	Topical anesthetic		Topical	To effect
Cetirizine	Antihistamine, allergies	0.15-5 mg/kg	PO	12
		5 mg/cat	PO	12
		2.5-10 mg/dog	PO	12-24
Charcoal, activated	See Activated charcoal			
Chlorambucil	Chronic lymphocytic leukemia	0.1-0.2 mg/kg (D)	PO	24-48
		2-6 mg/m^2 (D)	PO	24-48
		20 mg/m^2 (D)	PO	7-14 days
		0.25-0.5 mg/kg (C)	PO	48-72
		20 mg/m^2 (C)	PO	14-21 days
	Macroglobulinemia	Loading dose: 0.2 mg/kg (D)	PO	24 x 10 days with glucocorticoid
		Maintenance dose: 0.1 mg/kg	PO	24 with glucocorticoid
	Immune-mediated skin disease	0.1-0.2 mg/kg	PO	48 with glucocorticoid
	Lymphoplasmocytic enteritis	2-6 mg/m^2 (D)	PO	24-48
Chloramphenicol palmitate	*Susceptible bacterial infections	25-50 mg/kg (D)	PO	8
		50 mg/cat	PO	12

DRUG	INDICATIONS	DOSE	ROUTE	FREQUENCY (HR)
Chloramphenicol sodium succinate	*Susceptible bacterial infections	25-50 mg/kg (D)	IV, SC, IM	6-8
		50 mg/cat	IV, SC, IM	12
Chlordiazepoxide	Behavioral disorders	2.2-6.6 mg/kg	PO	PRN
	Behavioral disorders, anxiolytic	0.5-1 mg/kg (C)	PO	12-24
Chlordiazepoxide/ clidinium	Irritable colon syndrome	0.1-0.25 mg/kg (D). Based on clidinium dose	PO	8-12
Chlorhexidine acetate	Dental hygiene	Apply 0.10 mL solution topically	Topical	24
Chlorhexidine diacetate	Fungal skin infections	1 mL of 2% solution to 9 mL water	Topical	PRN
Chlorhexidine gluconate	Burns	Apply 0.5% solution after cleansing area	Topical	PRN
		Saturate wet dressing	Topical	12-24
	Dental hygiene	Apply 0.12% gel topically	Topical	24
Chlorothiazide	Diuretic	10-40 mg/kg	PO	12
	Partial antidiuretic hormone deficiency/diabetes insipidus (ADH)	20-40 mg/kg	PO	12
Chlorpheniramine maleate	Antihistamine	2-8 mg/dog	PO	8-12
		2-4 mg/dog	PO	12-24
	Behavioral disorders, excessive grooming, self-trauma	2-4 mg/dog	PO	12

DRUG	INDICATIONS	DOSE	ROUTE	FREQUENCY (HR)
continued—	Mild sedation	0.22 mg/kg (D)	PO	8-12
		1-2 mg/kg (C)	PO	8-12
Chlorpromazine hydro-chloride	Tranquilization	0.8-4.4 mg/kg (D)	PO	8-12
		0.5 mg/kg (C)	IM, IV	6-8
		2-4 mg/kg (C)	PO	24
	Antiemetic	0.5 mg/kg	IM, IV, SC	6-8
		0.05-0.5 mg/kg (D)	IM, SC	6-24
		1 mg/kg (D)	Per rectum	8
		3.3 mg/kg (D)	PO	6-24
		1.1-6.6 mg/kg (D)	IM	6-24
	Irritable colon syndrome	0.5 mg/kg (D)	IM	8-24
	Muscle relaxation during tetanus	0.5 mg/kg (D)	IM, IV	12
		2 mg/kg (D)	IM	12
	Preanesthetic	Maximum of 1.1 mg/kg (D)	IM	1-1.5 hours prior to surgery
	Prior to administration of anti-cancer drugs	2 mg/kg	SC	1 hour prior to therapy
	Amphetamine poisoning	10-18 mg/kg	IV	Once
Chlorpropamide	Partial antidiuretic hormone (ADH) deficiency/diabetes insipidus	10-40 mg/kg (D)	PO	24
Chlortetracycline	*Susceptible bacterial infections	25 mg/kg	PO	6-8

Drug	Indications	Dose	Route	Frequency (hr)
Cholecalciferol	See Vitamin D			
Cholestyramine	Short bowel syndrome	200-300 mg/kg	PO	12
		1-2 g/dog	PO	12
Chondroitin sulfate	Arthropathies (low molecular weight)	15-30 mg/kg	PO	24
Chorionic gonadotropin	Luteinize a follicular cyst	500-1,000 IU (D)	IM	2 doses, 48 h apart
	Induce descent of inguinal testis	25-100 IU	IM	2 x per week x 4-6 weeks
	Male hypogonadism	500 IU/dog	SC	2 x per week x 4 weeks then start pregnant mare serum (PMS)
	Induce ovulation	500-1,000 IU (D)	SC	24 x 2 days after administration of follicular stimulating hormone
		250 IU/cat	IM	On days 1 and 2 of estrus
Cimetidine	Esophagitis, gastric ulceration, antiemetic, chronic gastritis, GI tract ulceration	5-15 mg/kg	IM, IV, PO	6-12 (D), 8-12 (C). (See Appendix H)
	Gastrinemia	5-15 mg/kg	IV, PO, SC	6
	Effects of mast cell tumors	5 mg/kg (D)	IV, PO	6-8
	Immunomodulator	6-10 mg/kg	IM, IV, PO	8
Ciprofloxacin	*Susceptible bacterial infections	20-50 mg/kg (D)	IV, PO	12-24
		10-20 mg/kg (C)	IV	12-24

DRUG	INDICATIONS	DOSE	ROUTE	FREQUENCY (HR)
Cisapride	Prokinetic	0.1-0.5 mg/kg (D)	PO	8-12
		2.5-7.5 mg (C)	PO	8-12
Cisplatin	Anticancer	40-70 mg/m² (D)	IV	q 3 weeks with a saline solution as part of a protocol (See Appendix H)
Clarithromycin	*Susceptible bacterial infections	2.5-10 mg/kg (D)	PO	12-24
	Canine leproid granuloma syndrome	15-25 mg/kg	PO	Divide dose and administer q 8-12
	Leprosy	62.5 mg/cat	PO	12 with clofazimine
	Helicobacter	7.5 mg/kg (C)	PO	12 with metronidazole and amoxicillin
	M. tuberculosis-bovis	5-10 mg/kg	PO	12 with rifampin and enrofloxaxin
Clemastine	Antihistamine, allergic skin disease	0.05-0.5 mg/kg (D)	PO	12
		0.34-0.67 mg/cat	PO	12
	Atopy	0.15 mg/kg (C)	PO	12
Clindamycin	Anaerobic infections	5-11 mg/kg	PO	12
		22 mg/kg	PO	24
	Abscesses, dental infections	5.5-33 mg/kg	PO	12
	Stomatitis, acute pancreatitis	5-10 mg/kg	IM, IV	8
	Pancreatic exocrine insufficiency	5-10 mg/kg	PO	6-8, 30 min before meals
	Toxoplasmosis	12.5 mg/kg	IM, PO	12 x 28 days

32

Drug	Indications	Dose	Route	Frequency (hr)
continued –	Enteroepithelial cycle toxoplasmosis	12.5-50 mg/kg (C)	IM, PO	12
	Extraintestinal cycle toxoplasmosis	12.5-25 mg/kg (C)	IM, PO	12 x 2 weeks
	Hepatazoonosis	10 mg/kg (D)	PO	8 with pyrimethamine and trimethoprim/sulfa
Clofazimine	Feline leprosy	4-8 mg/kg	PO	24 x 6 weeks
		25-50 mg	PO	24 or 48
	Mycobacterium avium or *intracellularae* complex	4-8 mg/kg	PO	24 with doxycyline, clarithromycin, and/or enrofloxacin
Clomiphene citrate	Antiestrogen agent, infertility	25 mg/kg (D)	PO	24
Clomipramine	Behavioral disorders	1-3 mg/kg (D)	PO	12-24
		1-5 mg/cat	PO	12-24
		0.5-1 mg/kg (C)	PO	24
Clonazepam	Status epilepticus	1-10 mg/dog	PO	6-24
		50-200 μg/kg (D)	IV	To effect
	Adjunctive anticonvulsant	0.5-1.5 mg/kg (D)	PO	8-12
	Behavioral disorders, anxiolytic	0.05-0.25 mg/kg	PO	12-24
Clonidine	Growth hormone deficiency-diagnosis	10 μg/kg (D)	IV	Once

Drug	Indications	Dose	Route	Frequency (hr)
continued—	Refractory Diarrhea, inflammatory bowel disease	1-10 μg/kg (C)	PO, SC	8-12
Cloprostenol	Open cervix pyometra	1-5 μg/kg (D)	IM, SC	24 up to 21 days. Start with half dose and gradually increase over 2-3 days
	Abortifacient	1-2.5 μg/kg (D)	SC	24 x 4-7 days after 30 days of gestation
Clorazepate, sustained release	Behavioral disorders, fears, phobias	5.6 mg/small dog	PO	12-24
		11.25 mg/medium dog	PO	12-24
		22.5 mg/large dog	PO	12-24
		0.2-2.2 mg/kg (D)	PO	12-24
		0.2-0.5 mg/kg (C)	PO	12-24
Clorazepate dipotassium	Behavioral disorders, anxiolytic	1-2 mg/kg (C)	PO	8-12
	Anticonvulsant	0.5-2 mg/kg (D)	PO	8-12
Clotrimazole	Dermatophytosis	Apply to lesions	Topical	12 until culture is negative
	Antifungal	60 mL of 1 g/dL in polyethylene glycol	Topical (intranasal)	Over 1 h (under general anesthesia) repeat in 3-4 weeks PRN
Cloxacillin	*Susceptible bacterial infections	20-40 mg/kg	IM, IV, PO	4-8

Drug	Indications	Dose	Route	Frequency (hr)
Coal tar shampoos	Seborrhea		Topical	24. Keep in contact with skin for 10 min
Cobalamin	See Vitamin B12			
Cod liver oil	Hair coat (source of omega fatty acids)	5 mL (1 tsp)/10 kg	PO	24
Codeine	Cough	0.1-2 mg/kg (D)	PO	6-12
	Pain	0.5-4 mg/kg	PO	6-12
		1 mg with each 5 mg acetaminophen (Dog only)	PO	8-12
	Diarrhea	0.25-0.5 mg/kg (D)	PO	6-8
Codeine/acetaminophen	See Acetaminophen/with codeine			
Coenzyme Q	Dilated cardiomyopathy	30-90 mg/dog	PO	12
Colchicine	Chronic hepatic fibrosis	0.01-0.03 mg/kg (D)	PO	24
Colony stimulating factor	See Filgrastim			
Corticotropin gel	ACTH response test	0.5-2.2 IU/kg	IM	Once, pre-ACTH sample
Cortisone acetate	Hypoadrenocorticism	1 mg/kg	IM, PO	24
Cosyntropin	ACTH response test (alternative to corticotropin gel)	Pre-ACTH sample 0.005 mg/kg up to 0.25 mg (D)	IV	Once, pre-ACTH sample

DRUG	INDICATIONS	DOSE	ROUTE	FREQUENCY (HR)
continued—		Pre-ACTH sample 0.125 mg (C)	IV	Once, pre-ACTH sample
Cromolyn sodium 4%	Allergic conjunctivitis	Follow label instructions	Topical (ophthalmic)	Follow label instructions
Cyanocobalamin	See Vitamin B12		PO	24
Cyclizine	Antiemetic	4 mg/kg	IM	8
Cyclophosphamide	Anticancer	100 mg/m²	IV	See relevant protocols
	Immunosuppressive	2.2-4 mg/kg	PO	24 x 4 days per week or q 48
		50-100 mg/m²	PO	24 x 4 days per week or q 48
	Anticancer, immunosuppresive	6.25-12.5 mg (C)		24 x 4 consecutive days per week
	Feline infectious peritonitis	2-4 mg/kg (C)	PO	24 x 4 consecutive days per week
	Polymyositis	1 mg/kg (D)	PO	24 x 4 consecutive days per week
	Feline mammary cancer	100 mg/m² (C)	PO	Every 3 weeks with doxo-rubicin
	Multiple myeloma	7 mg/kg	IV	Once
	Eosinophilic enteritis	Initial dose: 6.6 mg/kg	PO	q 24 x 3 days
		Followed by: 2.2 mg/kg	PO	24
	Rheumatoid arthritis	<10 kg: 2.5 mg/kg (D)	PO	24 x 4 consecutive days per week
		10-35 kg: 2 mg/kg (D)	PO	24 x 4 consecutive days per week
		>35 kg: 1.8 mg/kg (D)	PO	24 x 4 consecutive days per week

36

DRUG	INDICATIONS	DOSE	ROUTE	FREQUENCY (HR)
Cylcosporine	Chronic allergic diseases	4-6 mg/kg	PO	12-48; monitor (See Appendix F)
	Immune-mediated diseases	4-10 mg/kg	PO	12; monitor (See Appendix F)
	Immune thrombocytopenia	4-6 mg/kg	4 hr IV infusion	12 (avoid extravasation)
	Systemic lupus erythematosus, sebaceous adenitis	5-20 mg/kg (D)	PO	12; monitor (See Appendix F)
	Perianal fistulas	1-7 mg/kg (D)	PO	12; monitor (See Appendix F)
Cyclosporine ophthalmic 1-2%	Keratoconjunctivitis sicca, pigmentary keratitis, plasmoma of third eyelid	Several drops	Topical (ophthalmic)	12
Cyproheptadine hydro-chloride	Antihistamine	1.1 mg/kg (D)	PO	8-12
	Appetite stimulant	2-4 mg/cat	PO	12-24
Cytarabine arabinoside	Anticancer	5-10 mg	IM, IV, SC	24 x 2 weeks
		30-50 mg/kg	IM, IV, SC	7 days
		100 mg/m²	IM, IV, SC	24 x 4 days (D) or q 2 days (C) then
		20 mg/m²	Intrathecal	24 x 1-5 days
Cythioate	Ectoparasites	1.5-3.3 mg/kg	PO	72 or 2 x per week
		1-30 mg tab/22 kg	PO	2 x per week
		0.22 mL/kg	PO	72 or 2 x week

Drug	Indications	Dose	Route	Frequency (HR)
Cytosine arabinoside	Lymphosarcoma, myeloproliferative disorders	100 mg/m²	IV	24 x 4 days
Dacarbazine	Lymphoreticular neoplasms	200-250 mg/m²	IV	24 x 5 days. Repeat every 21 days
	Soft tissue sarcomas	800-1,000 mg/m²	IV	Deliver entire dose over 6-8 hours or divide dose and administer 1 x per day x 5 days. Repeat q 21 days
Dactinomycin	Anticancer	0.015 mg/kg	IV	24 x 3-5 days. Repeat at 3 week intervals
		0.7-1.5 mg/m²	IV	7 days
		0.5-0.9 mg/m²	IV (over 20 min)	2-3 weeks
Dalteparin	Thromboembolic disease	100-150 IU/kg (D)	SC	8
		180 IU/kg (C)	SC	6
Danazol	Thrombocytopenia	5-10 mg/kg (D)	PO	12
		5 mg/kg (C)	PO	12
Dantrolene	Functional urethral obstruction	3-15 mg (D)	PO	8-12
		1-5 mg/kg (D)	PO	8
		0.5-2 mg/kg (C)	PO	8
Dapsone	Mycobacteriosis	0.3-1.1 mg/kg (D)	PO	8-12 for a minimum of 4-6 weeks (high dose until remission)

DRUG	INDICATIONS	DOSE	ROUTE	FREQUENCY (HR)
continued –		1 mg/kg (C)	PO	24 x 6 weeks
		12.5-25 mg/cat	PO	12-24
	Cutaneous vasculitis	1 mg/kg (D)	PO	8 x 14 days
	Subcorneal pustular dermatosis	1 mg/kg (D)	PO	8
	Brown recluse spider bite	0.7-1 mg/kg	PO	8
	Pemphigus	1 mg/kg	PO	8 (with sulfasalazine)
	Doxirubricin extravasation	1 mg/kg	PO	8
Decoquinate	Hepatazoonosis	10-20 mg/kg	PO	12 for 2 years
	To follow trimethoprim sulfa, clindamycin, and pyrimethamine therapy	10-20 mg/kg	PO	24
	Coccidiosis prophylaxis	50 mg/kg	PO	24
Deferoxamine mesylate	Iron chelator	Loading dose: 10 mg/kg	IM, IV, SC	2 x 2 doses
		Maintenance dose: 10 mg/kg	IM, IV, SC	8 x 3 treatments
	Cardiac arrest	5-15 mg/kg	IM, IV, SC	2 x 2 doses then 8 x 3 doses
		10 mg/kg	IM, IV	2 x 2 doses then 8 x 3 doses
	Reperfusion injuries	50 mg/kg	IV (over 5 min)	Once
Demeclocycline	Inappropriate antidiuretic hormone (ADH) secretion	3-12 mg/kg	PO	6-12
Deprenyl	See Selegiline			

DRUG	INDICATIONS	DOSE	ROUTE	FREQUENCY (HR)
Deracoxib	Antiinflammatory	1-2 mg/kg (D)	PO	24
	Postoperative analgesia	3-4 mg/kg (D)	PO	24 up to 7 days. Administer first dose night before surgery
Derm Caps	Skin disorders	1 capsule per 9 kg	PO	24
Derm Caps (liquid)	Skin disorders	<4.5 kg: 0.35 mL	PO	24
		4.5-8.9 kg: 0.7 mL	PO	24
		9-13.5 kg: 1.05 mL	PO	24
Derm Caps ES (liquid)	Skin disorders	<13.6 kg: 0.5 mL	PO	24
		13.6-27.1 kg: 1 mL	PO	24
		27.2-40.8 kg: 1.5 mL	PO	24
Desmopressin acetate (DDAVP)	von Willebrand's disease	1-4 μg/kg (D) diluted in saline	IV (over 15-30 min), SC	30 min prior to surgery
		0.3 μg/kg (diluted in 50 mL saline)	IV (over 15-30 min)	PRN
		Initial dose: 0.05-0.1 mg	PO	12 x 2 doses
		Followed by: 0.1-0.2 mg	PO	12
	Central diabetes insipidus	1-4 drops (2 μg of 0.1 mg/mL product)	SC, Topical (IN, subconjunctivally)	12-24
Desoxycorticosterone acetate	Hypoadrenocorticism	0.2-0.4 mg/kg. Maximum of 5 mg	IM	24
Desoxycorticosterone pivalate	Hypoadrenocorticism	25 mg IM (1 mg DOCA released/day)	IM	25 days
		125 mg pellet SC (0.5 mg DOCA released/day)	SC	6 months

Drug	Indications	Dose	Route	Frequency (hr)
continued−		1.5-2.2 mg/kg (D)	IM	25-28 days
		10-12.5/cat	IM	30 days
Dexamethasone	Cerebral edema, spinal cord	Initial dose: 2-3 mg/kg	IV	Once
		Maintenance dose: 0.1 mg/kg	IV	8-12
	Trauma, fibrocartilaginous disk, other CNS trauma	Loading dose: 1-2.2 mg/kg	IV, SC	Once
		Maintenance dose: 0.1 mg/kg	IV, PO, SC	8-12
	Hydrocephalus	0.25 mg/kg	IM, IV, PO	6-8
	Shock, anaphylaxis	4-6 mg/kg	IV (slowly)	Once
	Immune thrombocytopenia	Initial dose: 0.25-0.3 mg/kg (D)	IV, SC	Once
		Maintenance dose: 0.25-1.25 mg/kg	PO	12-24
		0.10-0.15 mg/kg	PO, SC	12 x 5-7 days then taper dose
	Adrenocortical collapse	0.1-0.5 mg/kg	IV, SC	With mineralocorticoids
	Asthma	Initial dose: 1 mg/kg	IV	Once
		Maintenance dose: 0.25-1 mg/cat	PO	8-24
Dexamethasone NaPO4	Shock	4-6 mg/kg	IV	Once
Dexpanthenol (pantothenic acid)	Intestinal atony	11 mg/kg	IM	4-6
Dexrazoxane	Iron chelation for doxorubicin-induced cardiotoxicity	25 mg/kg (ratio of 10-20:1 dexrazoxane-doxorubicin)	IV	15 min before doxorubicin

DRUG	INDICATIONS	DOSE	ROUTE	FREQUENCY (HR)
Dextran 40	Shock	10-20 mL/kg	IV	24
		2 mL/kg (in 5% D/W)	IV	24
	Frostbite	20-40 mL/kg (in 5% D/W)	IV	24
Dextran 70	Colloidal expansion	10-40 mL/kg	IV	24 to effect. (See Appendix H)
		10 mL/kg (C)	IV	24
Dextroamphetamine	Narcolepsy	5-10 mg	PO	8 (with imipramine)
	Hyperkinesis	0.2-1.3 mg/kg	PO	PRN
Dextromethorphan	Antitussive	0.5-2 mg/kg (D)	IV, PO, SC	6-8
	Combination analgesia, pruritis	2 mg/kg	IV, PO, SC	6-8
Dextrose 5%	Hypoglycemia, insulin overdosage	40-50 mL/kg	IP, IV, SC	PRN
Dextrose 50%	Hypoglycemia, insulin overdosage	2 mL/kg	PO	To effect
		0.25-1 mL/kg	IV	To effect
Diazepam	Restraint	0.2-0.6 mg/kg (D)	IV	To effect.
		0.25 mg	PO	8. Monitor. (See Appendix F)
	Sedation	0.5-2.2 mg/kg	PO	PRN
	Anticonvulsant	0.15-0.70 mg/kg (C)	PO	8
		2-5 mg/cat	PO	8

Drug	Indications	Dose	Route	Frequency (hr)
continued—		1-4 mg/kg (D)	PO	6-8
		2-5 mg/kg	IV, PO	8
		1-2 mg/kg	Per rectum	PRN
	Status epilepticus, certain toxicoses	0.5-5 mg/kg	IV	PRN. Start with a lower dose and increase in increments of 5-20 mg. (See Appendix H)
	Strychnine-induced seizures	2-5 mg/kg	IV	PRN
	Acquired tremors	0.25 mg/kg (D)	PO	6-8
	Scotty cramps	0.5-2 mg/kg (D)	IV, PO	To effect or q 8
	Preanesthetic	0.1-0.2 mg/kg (D)	IV (slowly)	
		0.22-0.44 mg/kg. Maximum of 5mg	IM, IV	To effect
		0.5 mg/kg	IV	To effect
	Irritable colon syndrome	0.15 mg/kg (D)	PO	8
	Reflex dyssynergia (urethral obstruction)	2.5-5 mg/cat	PO	6-8
		1.25-2.5 mg/cat	PO	8-12
		0.5 mg/kg	IV	To effect
	Appetite stimulant	0.05-0.4 mg/kg (C)	IM, IV, PO	24 or 48
		1 mg/cat	PO	24
	Functional urethral obstruction	2-10 mg	PO	8
	Behavioral disorders, psychogenic alopecia	1-2 mg/cat	PO	12
	Behavioral disorders	0.5-2.2 mg/kg (D)	PO	PRN

DRUG	INDICATIONS	DOSE	ROUTE	FREQUENCY (HR)
Diazoxide	Hypoglycemia	5-13 mg/kg (D). Maximum of 40 mg/kg	PO	Divide dose and administer q 8-12
Dichlorphenamide	Glaucoma	2-5 mg/kg (D)	PO	8-12
		10-12 mg/kg	PO	8-12
		0.5-1.5 mg/kg (C)	PO	8-12
Dichlorvos	Hookworms, whipworms, roundworms	11-22 mg/kg	PO	Once, repeat in 3 weeks if needed
		26-33 mg/kg (D)	PO	Once, repeat in 3 weeks if needed
		11 mg/kg (puppies)	PO	Once, repeat in 3 weeks if needed
		11 mg/kg (C)	PO	Once, repeat in 3 weeks if needed
Dicloxacillin	*Susceptible bacterial infections	30-50 mg/kg	PO	6-8
Dicoumarol	Anticoagulant	Initial dose: 5 mg/kg	PO	Once
		Maintenance dose: 1.3-2.6 mg/kg	PO	24
Dicyclomine	Detrusor hyperspasticity or urge incontinence	5-10 mg	PO	6-8
	Acute colitis, irritable colon	0.15 mg/kg (D)	PO	8

DRUG	INDICATIONS	DOSE	ROUTE	FREQUENCY (HR)
Dicycloverine	See Dicyclomine			
Diethylcarbamazine	Heartworm prophylaxis	6.6 mg/kg (D)	PO	24
	Roundworms	55-110 mg/kg	PO	24
Diethylstillbestrol	Hormone-responsive urinary incontinence	0.01-0.04 mg/kg	PO	24 x 7 days then 1-2 x per week
		0.1-1 mg (D)	PO	24 x 3-5 days then 1 x per week
	Feline symmetrical alopecia	0.625 mg/cat	PO	Once
	Testosterone-responsive tumors	0.02 mg/kg (D)	PO	24-48
		0.05-0.1 mg (C)	PO	24
	Estrogen-responsive dermatosis	0.02 mg/kg (D)	PO	24 x 14 days then q 48 x 3 months
	Mismating	0.1-1 mg/dog	PO	24 x 5 days starting 1-2 days postcoitus
		1-2 mg	PO	24 x 5 days after estradiol cyprionate therapy starting 5 days postcoitus
	Estrus induction	5 mg (D)	PO	24 x 7 days. If no response then
		10 mg (D)	PO	24 x 7
Difloxacin	*Susceptible bacterial infections	5-10 mg/kg	PO	24
Digitoxin	Heart failure, supraventricular tachyarrhythmias	0.03-0.1 mg/kg/day (D)	PO	Divide dose and administer q 8-12

DRUG	INDICATIONS	DOSE	ROUTE	FREQUENCY (HR)
continued—		0.005-0.015 mg/kg (C)	PO	24; monitor (See Appendix F)
		0.22 mg/m^2 (D)	PO (tablet)	12; monitor (See Appendix F)
		0.18 mg/m^2 (D)	PO (elixir)	12; monitor (See Appendix F)
Digoxin	Congestive heart failure	0.005-0.02 mg/kg (D)	PO (tablet)	12; monitor (See Appendix F)
		0.22 mg/m^2 (D)	PO (tablet)	12; monitor (See Appendix F)
	Supraventricular tachyarrhythmias	0.005-0.008 mg/kg/day (C)	PO (tablet)	Div. 12; monitor (See Appendix F)
		0.18 mg/m^2	IV, PO	If IV, give 25%-50% of dose q 1 h. If PO, administer q 12 hr
	Dilated cardiomyopathy	0.005-0.008 mg/kg (D)	PO (elixir)	12; monitor (See Appendix F)
		0.003-0.004 mg/kg (C)	PO (elixir)	12; monitor (See Appendix F)
		0.0055-0.011 mg/kg (D)	IV (Cardoxin)	Give 25%-50% of dose q 1 h
		2-3 kg: 0.0312 mg (C)	PO (Cardoxin)	48; monitor (See Appendix F)
		4-5 kg: 0.0312 mg (C)	PO (Cardoxin)	24-48; monitor (See Appendix F)
		>6 kg: 0.0312 mg (C)	PO (Cardoxin)	12; monitor (See Appendix F)
Dihydrostreptomycin	*Susceptible bacterial infections	20-30 mg/kg	IM, SC	24
	Leptospirosis, endocarditis, tuberculosis	10 mg/kg (D)	IM	6-12
	Brucellosis	3-5 mg/kg (D)	IM	12 (with minocycline)
	Yersinia pestis	10 mg/kg (C)	IM	6
		10-20 mg/kg (C)	IM	12

DRUG	INDICATIONS	DOSE	ROUTE	FREQUENCY (HR)
Dihydrotachysterol	Hypocalcemia with renal disease	0.125 mg/dog	PO	3 x per week
1, 25-dihydroxyvitamin D₃	See Vitamin D₃			
Diltiazem	Hypertension, hypertrophic cardiomyopathy, supraventricular tachyarrhythmias	0.125-0.35 mg/kg	IV (slowly)	q 15 min PRN to a total dose of 0.75 mg/kg. (See Appendix H)
	Acute atrial tachycardia	0.05-0.15 mg/kg	IV (slowly)	q 5 min PRN to a total dose of 0.1-0.3 mg/kg
		0.25 mg/kg	IV (slowly)	q 15 min PRN to a total dose of 0.75 mg/kg
		0.5-2 mg/kg	PO	8
		1.75-2.5 mg/kg (C)	PO	8
	Hypertrophic cardiomyopathy	7.5 mg (C)	PO	8-12
Diltiazem, extended-release (XR and Cardiazem CD)	See Diltiazem	1/2 of 60 mg tablet or 10 mg/kg (C) Cardizem	PO	24
		30 mg (C) extended release	PO	24
Dimenhydrinate	Motion sickness	25-50 mg/dog	PO	8-24
		12.5 mg/cat	PO	8
		4-8 mg/kg	PO	8
Dimercaprol (BAL)	Arsenic toxicosis	2.5-5 mg/kg	IM	4 x 12 doses then q 8 x 3 doses then q 12

DRUG	INDICATIONS	DOSE	ROUTE	FREQUENCY (HR)
Dimethyl sulfoxide 40%	Spinal cord trauma	0.5-1 g/kg (D). Dilute to a 10% solution	IV (over 45 min)	6-8
Diminazene aceturate	Babesiosis, trypanosomiosis, cytauxzoonosis	3.5-10 mg/kg (D)	IM, SC	24
		2 mg/kg	IM, SC	96
		2-3.5 mg/kg	IM	Once
Dinoprost tromethamine	See Prostaglandin F_2 alpha			
Dioctyl sulfosuccinate	Stool softener	25 mg/small dog or cat	PO	12-24
		50-100 mg/medium or large dog	PO	12-24
Diphemanil methylsulfate	Parasympatholytic (bradycardia)	1.8 mg/kg	IM	12
Diphenhydramine	Antihistamine	2-4 mg/kg	PO	6-8
	Mast cell disease, antiemetic	2 mg/kg	IM, IV (slowly)	12 or PRN
	Anaphylaxis, urticaria	2 mg/kg	IM, IV (slowly)	12 or PRN
	Angioneurotic edema	2 mg/kg	IM, IV (slowly)	12 or PRN
	Antipruritic, allergic skin disease	1-2 mg/kg (D)	PO	8-12
		5-50 mg	IM	12
Diphenoxylate (contains atropine)	Acute colitis, irritable colon syndrome	0.1-0.2 mg/kg (D)	PO	8
		0.05-0.2 mg/kg (C)	PO	12

Drug	Indications	Dose	Route	Frequency (hr)
continued—	Antidiarrheal	2.5-10 mg (D)	PO	8
		0.6-1.2 mg (C)	PO	8-12
	Antitussive	0.2-0.5 mg (D)	PO	12
Diphenylhydantoin	See Phenytoin			
Diphenylthiocarbazone	Thallium toxicosis	50-70 mg/kg	PO	8
Dipyridamole	Antithrombotic	4-10 mg/kg	PO	24
Dipyrone	Antipyretic	25-100 mg/kg (D)	IM, IV, PO, SC	8
		25 mg/kg (C)	IM, IV, PO, SC	8 (low dose); 12-24 (high dose)
Dirlotapide	Weight loss	0.1 ml/kg (D)	PO	24 x 14 days
		0.2 ml/kg (D)	PO	24 x 14 days then base on current weight (see package insert)
Disodium EDTA	See Edetate disodium			
Disophenol	Hookworms	10 mg/kg (0.22 mL/kg) (D)	SC	Once then repeat in 2-3 weeks
	Spirocercosis	7.7 mg/kg (D)	SC	Once then repeat in 7 days
Disopyramide PO4	Ventricular dysrhythmias	6-22 mg/kg (D)	PO	8 (12 if long-acting product)
Dithiazanine iodide	Microfilaricide	6.6-11 mg/kg	PO	24 x 7-10 days
Divalproex sodium	See Valproic acid			

DRUG	INDICATIONS	DOSE	ROUTE	FREQUENCY (HR)
DL methionine	See Methionine			
Dobutamine	Inotropic agent	5-20 μg/kg (D)	CRI	(See Appendix H)
		2.5-15 μg/kg (C)	CRI (caution)	(See Appendix H)
Docusate calcium, sodium	Stool softener	25-200 mg (D)	PO	12
		50 mg/cat	PO	12-24
Dolasetron mesylate	Antiemetic	0.6 mg/kg	IV, PO, SC	24
Domperidone	Prokinetic agent, antiemetic	2 mg/kg	PO	12-24
		0.1-0.3 mg/kg	IM, IV, PO	12
Dopamine hydrochloride	Inotropic agent	2-25 μg/kg. Up to 50 μg/kg if severe hypotension or shock	CRI	(See Appendix H)
	Renal vasodilator: (acute renal failure)	2-5 μg/kg (low dose) in 5% D/W	CRI	(See Appendix H)
	Acute heart failure	2-10 μg/kg (40 mg in 500 mL)	CRI	(See Appendix H)
Doramectin	Susceptible ectoparasites (demodectic, sarcoptic mange)	600 μg/kg	SC	7 days x 4 weeks
Doxapram	Respiratory stimulant	1-5 mg/kg	IV	PRN
	Neonate	1-2 drops	Sublingual	To effect
		0.1 mL or 10 mg/m^2	IV (umbilical vein)	To effect
Doxepin	Behavior modification	3-5 mg/kg (D). Maximum of 150 mg	PO	12
	Pruritis	0.5-1 mg/kg	PO	12

Drug	Indications	Dose	Route	Frequency (hr)
Doxorubicin	Antineoplastic	> 20 kg: 30 mg/m²-250 mg/m² (D)	IV	21 days
		≤ 20 kg: 1 mg/kg (D);	IV	21 days
		10 mg/m² or 1.25 mg/kg (C)	IV	21 days
		20-30 mg/m² (C)	IV	21-28 days
Doxycyline	*Susceptible bacterial infections	5-10 mg/kg	IV, PO	12-24
	Salmon poisoning	10 mg/kg	IV	12
	Ehrlichia, Rocky Mountain Spotted Fever	5 mg/kg	IV, PO	12
	Haemobartenellosis	5 mg/kg	PO	12
	Bartonellosis	50 mg	PO	12
	Toxoplasmosis	5-10 mg/kg	PO	12-24
Doxylamine succinate	Antihistamine	1.1-2.2 mg/kg	IM, PO, SC	8-12
D-Penicillamine	See Penicillamine			
Edetate (EDTA) calcium	Lead poisoning	25-100 mg/kg of a 1% solution (mix 1 g in 100 mL 5% D/W). Maximum of 2 g	SC	6 x 5 days
Edetate (EDTA) disodium	Calcium keratopathy	0.37% solution	Topical (lavage cornea)	Lavage for 15-20 min q 12 h cornea
		1% solution 1-2 drops	Topical	12 x several weeks
Edrophonium	Tensilon test	0.11-0.22 mg/kg (D). Maximum of	IV	Once

DE

DRUG	INDICATIONS	DOSE	ROUTE	FREQUENCY (HR)
continued—		5 mg		
		0.1-0.5 mg/puppy	IV	Once
		0.25-0.5 mg/cat	IV	Once
Emetine	Emesis	1-2.5 mL/kg (D). Maximim of 6.6 mL/kg	PO	Once
		3.3 mL/kg, dilute 50:50 with water (C)	PO	Once
Emodepside/praziquantel	Susceptible endoparasites	0.35-1.12 mL (C)	Topical	Monthly
Enalapril	Hypertension, heart failure, valvular insufficiency	0.2-1 mg/kg (D)	PO	12-24
	Progressive renal disease	0.25-0.5 mg/kg (C)	PO	12-24
Endotoxin antisera	Endotoxemia	4-8 mg/kg	IV	Once
Enflurane	Anesthesia	Induction: 2%-3%		
		Maintenance: 1.5%-3.0%		
Enilconazole	Nasal aspergillosis	5% solution	Topical (instill into nasal sinus)	12 x 7-10 days
		10-20 mg/kg (10% solution diluted 50:50 with water)	Topical (instill into nasal sinus)	12 x 10-14 days
	Dermatophytes	Dilute to 0.2% solution	Wash affected area	72-96 x 4 treatments
Enoxaparin	Thromboembolic disease	0.8 mg/kg (D)	SC	6
		1.25 mg/kg (C)	SC	6

Drug	Indications	Dose	Route	Frequency (hr)
Enrofloxacin	*Susceptible bacterial infections	5-20 mg/kg	IM, IV, PO, SC	12-24
	Pseudomonas infections	20 mg/kg	PO	12
		5 mg/kg (C)	PO	24
Ephedrine	Bronchodilator, decongestant	2-5 mg/cat	PO	8-12
		1-2 mg/kg (D)	PO	8-12
	Urinary incontinence	4 mg/kg (D) or 12.5-50 mg/dog	PO	8-12
		2-4 mg/kg (C)	PO	8-12
		0.25 tablet/cat	PO	4-6
Epinephrine		Use 1:10,000 (0.1 mg/mL)	Dilute 1 mL in 10 mL saline to make 1:1000 (0.01 mg/mL or 10 μg/mL)	
	Cardiac Arrest	10-20 μg/kg	IV	PRN every 5-15 min
		200 μg/kg	IV	PRN every 5-15 min
		0.8-2 mg/kg	IT	PRN every 5-15 min
	Anaphylaxis	0.1- 0.2 mL/kg (0.01-0.02 mg/kg)	IM, IV, SC	PRN every 5-15 min
		2.5-5 μg/kg	IV	PRN every 5-15 min
		50 μg/kg	IT	PRN every 5-15 min
	Asthma	0.1 mL/kg	IM, IV, SC	PRN every 5-15 min
		0.1 mg (1 ml) (C)	IM, IV, SC	PRN every 5-15 min
Epoetin	See Erythropoietin			

DRUG	INDICATIONS	DOSE	ROUTE	FREQUENCY (HR)
Epsiprantel	Tapeworms (*Dipylidium*, *Taenia*)	5-5.5 mg/kg (D)	PO	Once
		2.5-2.75 mg/kg (C)	PO	Once
Ergocalciferol	See Vitamin D2			
Erythromycin	*Susceptible bacterial infections	10-22 mg/kg (D). Maximum of 40 mg/kg	PO	8-12
		10-22 mg/kg (C)	IV, PO	8
		3-5 mg/kg (C)	IM	8
Erythropoietin	Anemia from renal failure	50-100 Units/kg	IV, SC	3 x per week x 12 weeks then 2 x per week PRN to maintain hematocrit >35%
Erythropoietin	Anemia from renal failure	400 Units/kg	IV, SC	Once per week (adjust to maintain a hematocrit of 30-34%)
Esmolol	Selective B1 blockade, ventricular arrythmias	0.05-0.1 mg/kg (D)	IV (slow bolus)	q 5 min to a total cumulative dose of 0.5 mg/kg
		Loading dose: 200-500 µg/kg	IV (slow bolus)	Once
		Maintenance dose: 25-200 µg/kg	CRI	(See Appendix H)
Essential fatty acids	See Derm Caps			
Estradiol cypionate	Mismating, estrus induction, replacement	20-44 µg/kg (D). Maximum of 1 mg	IM	Once during estrus or within 72 hours of mismating

54

Drug	Indications	Dose	Route	Frequency (hr)
continued—		125-250 μg/cat	IM	Once between 40 hours and 5 days after mismating
Ethacrynic acid	Diuretic, pulmonary edema	0.2-0.4 mg/kg	IM, IV	4-12
Ethambutol	Tuberculosis	15 mg/kg (D)	PO	24
		25 mg/kg (D)	PO	72
Ethanol 20%	Ethylene glycol toxicosis	5.5 mL/kg (D)	IV	4 x 5 treatments then q 6 x 4 treatments. (See Appendix H)
		5 mL/kg (C)	IV	6 x 5 treatments then q 8 x 4 treatments
Ethosuximide	Seizures	Loading dose: 40 mg/kg	PO	Once
		Maintenance dose: 20 mg/kg	PO	
Ethoxzolamide	Glaucoma	4 mg/kg (D)	PO	12
Ethylisobutrazine hydrochloride	Sedation	4.4-11 mg/kg (D)	IM, PO	PRN
		2.2-4.4 mg/kg (D)	IV	PRN
Etidronate disodium	Hypercalcemia associated with neoplastic disease	5-20 mg/kg	PO	24
Etodolac	Antiinflammatory, osteoarthritis	5-15 mg/kg (D)	PO	24
Etomidate	Anesthetic induction	0.5-2 mg/kg	IV	To effect

DRUG	INDICATIONS	DOSE	ROUTE	FREQUENCY (HR)
Etomidate with opioids	Anesthetic induction	0.5-1 mg/kg	IV	To effect
Etretinate	Primary seborrhea	0.75-1 mg/kg (D)	PO	24
	All other dermatologic indications	1-2 mg/kg/day (C)	PO	24
Euthanasia solution with pentobarbital	Euthanasia	120 mg/kg for the first 4.5 kg and 60 to 120 mg/kg thereafter	IV	To effect
Euthanasia solution (T-61)	Euthanasia	0.66 mL/kg (D)	IV	To effect
		1-10 mL (C)	IV	To effect
Famotidine	Gastric ulcers, esophagitis	0.5-1 mg/kg (D)	IM, IV, PO, SC	12-24
Febantel	Susceptible endoparasites	10 mg/kg	PO	24 x 3 days (with 1 mg/kg praziquantel)
		15 mg/kg (puppies)	PO	24 x 3 days
Felbamate	Anticonvulsant	15-65 mg/kg (D). Maximum of 200 mg (small) and 400 mg (large)	PO	8-12 PRN
Fenbendazole	*Paragonimus kellicotti*	25-50 mg/kg	PO	12 x 10-14 days
	Aelurostrongylus abstrusus	25-50 mg/kg (C)	PO	12 x 10-14 days
	Capillaria aerophilia sp.	25-55 mg/kg/day (D)	PO	12 (low dose) - 24 (high dose) x 3-14 days depending or organism
	Capillaria aerophilia sp.	25-55 mg/kg/day (C)	PO	24 x 10-14 days

DRUG	INDICATIONS	DOSE	ROUTE	FREQUENCY (HR)
continued –	*Capillaria feliscati* sp.	25 mg/kg (C)	PO	12 x 3 days
	Capillaria plica sp.	50 mg/kg	PO	24 x 3. Repeat in 3 weeks
	Crenosoma vulpis, Guardia	50 mg/kg (D)	PO	24 x 3 days
	Eucoleus boehmi	50 mg/kg (D)	PO	24 x 10-14 days
	Eurytrema procyonic	30 mg/kg (C)	PO	24 x 3 days
	Filaroides hirthi	Start at 30 mg/kg, gradually increase to 65 mg/kg	PO	24 x 10-14 days
	Giardiosis	50 mg/kg (D)	PO	24 x 3-7 days
	Hookworms, whipworms, roundworms and tapeworms (*Taenia* only)	50 mg/kg (C)	PO	24 x 3-5 days. Repeat in 3 weeks
	Prevention of transplacental and transmammary transmission	50-55 mg/kg	PO	24 from 40th day of pregnancy to 14th day of lactation
Fentanyl citrate	Analgesia	Loading dose: 5 μg/kg (D)	IV	Once
		Maintenance dose: 3-10 μg/kg (D)	CRI	(See Appendix H)
		Loading dose: 2-3 μg/kg (C)	IV	Once
		Maintenance dose: 2-3 μg/kg (C)	CRI	(See Appendix H)
	Perioperative pain	5-10 μg/kg (D)	IM, IV, CRI, SC	(See Appendix H)
		2.5-5 μg/kg (C)	IV, CRI	(See Appendix H)
	Induction	1-5 μg/kg (D)	IV	To effect
		1-2 μg/kg (C)	IV	To effect
	Transdermal patch	0.01 mg/kg	Transdermal	2-5 days (approximate)

DRUG	INDICATIONS	DOSE	ROUTE	FREQUENCY (HR)
continued—		25 μg/hr (C)	Transdermal	2-5 days (approximate)
		<10 kg: 25 μg/hr	Transdermal	2-5 days (approximate)
		10-20 kg: 50 μg/hr	Transdermal	2-5 days (approximate)
		20-30 kg: 75 μg/hr	Transdermal	2-5 days (approximate)
		>30 kg: 75 μg/hr	Transdermal	2-5 days (approximate)
Fentanyl/droperidol	Tranquilization	>25 kg: 75 μg/hr	IV	To effect
		0.3-0.5 mL/55 kg (D)	IV	To effect
		0.04-0.09 mL/kg (D)	IM	To effect
		0.01-0.14 mL/kg (D)	IM	To effect
	Preanesthetic	0.11 mL/kg (C)	IM	To effect
Fenthion (Pro Spot 10) 5.6%	Fleas	0.5 mL/kg (D)	Topical	14 days
		0.35 mL/4.5 kg (C)	Topcial	14 days
Ferric cyanoferrate	Thallium toxicosis	4-8 mg/kg	PO	8
Ferrous sulfate	Dietary iron supplement	100 mg/kg	PO	24
		100-300 mg/dog	PO	24
		50-100 mg/cat	SC	24 (D) 12 (C)
Fexofenadine	Allergies, antihistamine	30 mg/kg (D)	PO	12
Filgrastim (granulocyte-colony stimulating factor; G-CSF)	Neutropenia	1-5 μg/kg (C)	SC	12-24
		3-10 μg/kg (C)	SC	24
		1-5 μg/kg (D)	SC	24

DRUG	INDICATIONS	DOSE	ROUTE	FREQUENCY (HR)
Finasteride	Antitestosterone: benign prostatic hypertrophy	1-5 µg/kg	PO	24
Fipronil	Susceptible ectoparasites	0.67-4 mL of 9.7% (D)	Topical	2-3 months
	Fleas, Ticks, Lice, Mites	0.5 mL of 9.7% (C)	Topical	Monthly
Fipronil with methoprene	Fleas, ticks, flea larvae	0.67-4 mL of 9.7% fipronil and 8.8% (S)-methoprene (D)	Topical	Monthly
	As above	0.5 mL of 9.7% fipronil, 8.8% (S)-methoprene (C)	Topical	Monthly
Firocoxib	Antiinflammatory, osteoarthritis	5 mg/kg (D)	PO	24
	Postoperative pain	5 mg/kg (D)	PO	24 x 3 days
Flavoxate	Detrusor hyperspasticity, urge incontinence	5 mg/kg (D)	PO	6-8
Florfenicol	*Susceptible bacterial infections	100-200 mg	IM, PO, SC	8 (D), 12 (C)
		25-50 mg/kg	PO, SC	8
		20 mg/kg (D)	IM, PO	12
		22 mg/kg (C)	IM, PO	6-8
Fluconazole	Blastomycosis	5 mg/kg	PO	12
	Cryptococcosis	2.5-10 mg/kg	PO (with food)	12-24
		150-200 mg/cat	PO	24 or divide dose and administer q 8

F

DRUG	INDICATIONS	DOSE	ROUTE	FREQUENCY (HR)
Flucytosine (combination therapy)	Cryptococcosis	125-250 mg/cat	PO	Divide dose and administer q 6-8. Do not use as sole therapy
		150-175 mg/kg	PO	Divide dose and administer q 6-8
		25-50 mg/kg	PO	6
	Urinary candidiasis	50-75 mg/kg. Maximum of 100 mg/kg	PO	8. Alkalinize urine to > 7.4
Fludrocortisone	Hypoadrenocorticism	0.01-0.02 mg/kg	PO	24. Adjust dose by increments of 0.05-0.1 mg
		0.05-0.1 mg/cat	PO	24
Flumazenil	Hepatic encephalopathy	0.01-0.02 mg	IV	PRN
Flumethasone	Antiinflammatory	0.1 mg/kg	IM, IV, PO, SC	24
		0.06-0.25 mg/dog	IA	Once
		0.166-1 mg	Intralesional	Once
Flunixin meglumine	Antiinflammatory	0.125-1 mg	IV	12-24 x 3 treatments
	Acute gastric dilatation, shock	0.5-2.2 mg/kg	IM, IV, SC	24 x 3 days maximum
	Gastrointestinal tract obstruction	1 mg/kg (D)	IV	12-24 x 3 treatments
	Acral lick dermatitis	0.5 mg/kg (D)	Topical (Synotic)	8-12
	Ocular	0.25 mg/kg	IM, IV, SC	12-24 x 5 treatments

DRUG	INDICATIONS	DOSE	ROUTE	FREQUENCY (HR)
5-Fluorouracil	Anticancer	0.25-0.5 mg/kg (D)	IV	q 7 days. Contraindicated in cats
		150 mg/m^2(D)	PO	24
Fluoxetine hydrochloride	Behavioral disorders, separation anxiety	1-2 mg/kg (D)	PO	24
	Behavioral disorders, stereotypic behavior	1-2 mg/kg (D)	PO	24
		1-3 mg/kg (D)	PO	24
		0.5-5 mg/cat	PO	24
Fluoxymesterone	Testosterone-responsive dermatosis	10 mg/kg	PO	48 x 12 weeks
Flurazepam	Appetite stimulant	0.5 mg/kg (D). Maximum of 30 mg/day	PO	4-7 days
Flurbiprofen	Allergic conjunctivitis	0.2-0.4 mg/kg	Topical	8-12
Fluticasone proprionate	Asthma	222 μg (1 puff)	Metered dose inhaler	12 to 24 or to effect
Fluvoxamine	Behavioral disorders	0.5-2 mg/kg (D)	PO	12
		0.25-0.5 mg/kg (C)	PO	24
Folic acid	Nutritional supplement	0.25-0.5 mg/kg (C)	PO	24
	Supplement to pyrimethamine	2.5 mg/cat	PO	24
Folinic acid (leucovorin)	Rescue for sulfonamides	1 mg/kg	PO	24

DRUG	INDICATIONS	DOSE	ROUTE	FREQUENCY (HR)
continued—	Rescue for methotrexate	3 mg/m^2	IM, IV, PO	Within 3 h of each methotrexate administration
Follicle stimulating hormone	Induction of estrus	20 IU/kg (D) (1 IU = 9.4-14.2 mg)	SC	24 x 10 days then
		500 IU Human Chorionic Gonadotropin	SC	24 x 2 days
		100 IU Pregnant Mare Serum (C)	SC	Once, then
		25-50 IM Pregnant Mare Serum	SC	24 x 7 days, then
		2 mg FSH	IM	24 x 3-5 days
	Male hypogonadism	2 mg FSH-P/cat	SC	3 x per week
Fomepizole	See 4-methylpyrazole			
Formoterol	Bronchodilation	1-3 puffs	Metered dose inhaler	12 to 24
Formoterol/budesonide	See Formoterol			
Foscarnet sodium	Susceptible viral infections	20-30 mg/kg (D)	IV, PO	8
Furazolidone	Giardiosis	4 mg/kg	PO	12 x 7-10 days
	Amoebic colitis	2.2 mg/kg (D)	PO	8 x 7 days
	Cystoisospora spp	8-20 mg/kg	PO	12-24 x 5 days
	Entamebiasis	2.2 mg/kg	PO	8 x 7 days
	Coccidiosis	8-20 mg/kg	PO	24 x 5 days
Furosemide	Diuresis with acute renal failure	5-20 mg/kg	IM, IV, PO	8-12 or PRN. Adjust to lowest dose possible
	Hypertension	1-2 mg/kg. Maximum of 8 mg/kg for acute renal failure	PO	12

DRUG	INDICATIONS	DOSE	ROUTE	FREQUENCY (HR)
continued—	Hydrocephalus, brain edema	0.5-2 mg/kg	PO	12
	Ascites from hepatic failure	1-2 mg/kg	PO, SC	12-24
	Hypercalcemia	1-2 mg/kg	IM, IV, PO, SC	8-12
		5 mg/kg	IV	PRN
		2-5 mg/kg	IV	To effect
		0.1-1 mg/kg	CRI	(See Appendix H)
Gabapentin	Anticonvulsant	10-30 mg/kg	PO	8
	Analgesic adjuvant, cancer pain	3 mg/kg	PO	24
	Analgesic, neuropathic pain	10-30 mg/kg (D)	PO	8
Gamma globulin	Immune-mediated disease	300-1,200 mg (D)	IV	6-12
Gemfibrozil	Hyperlipidemia	7.5 mg/kg	PO	12
Gentamicin	*Susceptible bacterial infections	6-8 mg/kg	IV, IM, SC	24
		4-8 mg/kg (D). Apply light coating	Topical	24; consider monitoring (See Appendix F)
Glargine insulin	See Insulin, glargine			
Glimepiride	Noninsulin-dependent diabetes mellitus	1-2 mg/cat	PO	24
Glipizide	Noninsulin-dependent diabetes mellitus	2.5-5 mg/cat	PO (with food)	12

DRUG	INDICATIONS	DOSE	ROUTE	FREQUENCY (HR)
Glucagon	Hypoglycemia (for transient control of)	Initial dose: 50 ng/kg	IV (bolus)	Once
		Followed by: 10-15 ng/kg. Maximum of 40 ng/kg	CRI	(See Appendix H)
	Hypoglycemia associated with insulinoma	5 ng/kg	CRI	(See Appendix H)
Glucose 40% ophthalmic	Corneal edema, nonhealing erosions	Apply 0.3 cm long strip	Topical	2-6 x per day
Glucosamine hydrochloride	Arthritis	20 mg/kg	PO	24
Glucosamine sulfate	Arthritis	40 mg/kg	PO	24
	Gastrointestinal inflammation	0.5 g/kg	PO	24
Glyburide	Noninsulin-dependent diabetes mellitus	0.625 mg/cat. Maximum of 2.5 mg/cat	PO	24
Glycerin	Acute glaucoma	0.5-2 ml/kg	PO	Repeat once at 8 hrs
Glycerin, enema	Constipation/obstipation	250 mg or 12 mL glycerin	Per rectum	1; repeat once only
Glyceryl guaiacolate	See Guaifenesin			
Glyceryl monoacetate	Sodium fluoroacetate toxicosis	0.55 mg/kg. Maximum of 2-4 mg/kg	IM	Hourly until maximum dose reached
Glycopyrrolate	Sinus bradycardia, SA block, AV block	0.005-0.010 mg/kg	IM, IV	PRN
		0.01-0.02 mg/kg	SC	8-12

G

Drug	Indications	Dose	Route	Frequency (hr)
continued—	Hypersialism	0.01 mg/kg	SC	PRN
	Preanesthetic	0.01-0.02 mg/kg	IM, SC	PRN
Gold sodium thiomalate	Challenge test	125-250 ng/kg	IM	Once
	Immune-mediated disease	1-5 mg	IM	Once in the first week
		2-10 mg	IM	Once in the second week
		1 mg/kg	IM	q 7 days (maintenance)
Gonadotropin-releasing hormone	Ovarian follicular cyst	50-100 µg	IM	1-3 treatments
	Stimulate ovulation	50 µg/dog	IV	1-3 treatments
		25 µg/cat	IM	After mating or on day 2 of estrus
	Undescended testes	50-100 µg/dog	IV, SC	Once. If no response repeat in 4-6 days
Gonadotropin, chorionic	Induce ovulation	22 IU/kg (D)	IM	Once
		44 IU/dog	IM	Once
	Luteinization of follicles	500-1000 IU	IM	Repeat in 48 h
	Hypogonadism	500 IU	SC	2 x per week for 4 weeks
	Descent of inguinal testicles	25-100 IU	IM	2 x per week for 4-6 weeks
Granisetron	Antiemetic	0.01 mg/kg	IV, PO	PRN
Graunlocyte-colony stimulating factor	See Filgrastim			

Drug	Indications	Dose	Route	Frequency (hr)
Griseofulvin (microsize)	Dermatophytosis	10-30 mg/kg	PO (with fatty meal)	24 or divide dose and administer q 8-12
		50 mg/kg	PO (with fatty meal)	24 or divide dose and administer q 8-12
		80-130 mg/kg	PO (with fatty meal)	24 or divide dose and administer q 8-12
Griseofulvin (ultramicrosize)		5-10 mg/kg	PO	24
		20-50 mg/kg	PO	24
Growth hormone (somatotropin)	Adult hyposomatotropism	0.1 IU/kg or 0.5 mg/kg (D)	SC	48 x 30 days
	Pituitary dwarfism	0.1 IU/kg or 0.5 mg/kg (D)	SC	24 x 3 days per week x 4-6 weeks
Guaifenesin	Restraint in dogs as sole agent	44-88 mg/kg	IV	To effect
	Restraint in dogs with thiamylal	33-88 mg/kg	IV	To effect
	Restraint in dogs with ketamine (1.1 mg/kg)	33-88 mg/kg	IV	To effect
	Muscle relaxation in cases of toxicoses (e.g., strychnine or tetanus)	110 mg/kg (D)	IV	PRN
Halothane	Anesthesia	Induction: 3%	Inhalant	To effect
		Maintenance: 0.5-1.5%	Inhalant	To effect

DRUG	INDICATIONS	DOSE	ROUTE	FREQUENCY (HR)
Hemoglobin (polymerized bovine)	Blood replacement	10-30 mL/kg	IV	Once. Maximum of 10 mL/hr
	Hypovolemic shock, as colloid	3-5 mL/kg with crystalloid at 0.5-2 x maintenance	IV	PRN. Monitor APTT to 1.5-2 times pretreatment baseline
Heparin	Arterial thromboembolism, thrombophlebitis	Initial dose: 100-200 IU/kg. Maximum of 500 IU/kg (D)	IV	Once
		Initial dose: 375 IU/kg (C)	IV	Once
		Maintenance dose: 100-300 IU/kg	SC	6-8
	Prophylaxis	Low dose: 10-50 IU/kg	SC	8-12
	Feline thromboembolism associated with cardiomyopathy	Induction: 1,000 IU/kg	IV	Once
		Maintenance: 50 IU/kg	SC	8
	During acute pancreatitis	50-100 IU/kg	SC	8-12
	Disseminated Intravascular Coagulation	75-100 IU/kg	IV, SC	6-8
		5,000 IU/500 mL blood	IV	PRN
	Low dose	5-10 IU/kg	IV infusion	Hourly. (See Appendix H)
	Burns	100-200 IU/kg	IV, SC	8 x 1-4 treatments
	Closed chest lavage	1,000 IU/L fluid at 20 mL/kg	Intrathoracic	12
	Lipoprotein lipase provocative test	100 IU/kg	IV	Test lipids before and 15 min after heparin

DRUG	INDICATIONS	DOSE	ROUTE	FREQUENCY (HR)
Heparin, low molecular weight	See Dalteperin			
Hetacillin	*Susceptible bacterial infections	20-44 mg/kg	PO on an empty stomach	8-12
		50 mg/cat	PO	12
Hetastarch	See Hydroxyethyl starch			
Human gamma globulin	Immunosuppression	0.5-1.5 g/kg	IV over 12 hr	Once
Hyaluronate sodium	Synovitis	3-5 mg	IA	7 days
Hydralazine	Vasodilator, heart failure	Initial dose: 0.5 mg/kg	PO	Once
		Then titrate up to: 1-3 mg/kg (D)	PO	12
		0.5-0.8 mg/kg (C)	PO	12
	Hypertension	0.5-2.0 mg/kg (D)	PO	8-12
		2.5 mg/cat	PO	12
	Acute arterial thromboembolism	0.5-2 mg/kg (D)	IM, PO	12
		2.5 mg/cat. Maximum of 10 mg/cat	PO	12
Hydrochlororthiazide	Diuretic	2-4 mg/kg (D)	PO	24
	Antihypertensive agent	0.5-2 mg/kg	PO	12-24
	Nephrogenic diabetes insipidus	0.5-5 mg/kg	PO	12
	Hypoglycemia	2-4 mg/kg (D)	PO	12 (with diazoxide)
		2-4 mg/kg	PO	12
	Calcium oxalate uroliths	2 mg/kg	PO	12

DRUG	INDICATIONS	DOSE	ROUTE	FREQUENCY (HR)
Hydrocodone bitartrate	Antitussive	0.25 mg/kg. Maximum of 1 mg/kg (D)	PO	6-8
		2.5-5 mg/cat	PO	8-12. Use with caution
Hydrocortisone	Replacement therapy	0.5-1 mg/kg	PO	24
	Antiinflammatory	2.5-5 mg/kg	PO	12
Hydrocortisone aurate	Hypoadrenocorticism	0.1-0.2 mg/kg	IM	8-12
	Immune-mediated hemolytic-anemia	2-4 mg/kg	IM	12-24
Hydrocortisone sodium succinate	Antiinflammatory	5-8 mg/kg	IV	12-24
	Shock	50-150 mg/kg	IV	8 x 2 treatments
	Hypoadrenocortical crisis	5-20 mg/kg (D)	IV	2-6
Hydrogen peroxide 3%	Emetic	5-10 mL	PO	Repeat once in 20-30 minutes
Hydromorphone	Analgesia	0.05-0.3 mg/kg	IM, IV, SC	2-6
	Preoperative medication	0.1 mg/kg	IM, IV, SC	To effect
	Alternative induction medication	0.1-0.2 mg/kg	IV infusion	To effect. (See Appendix H)
Hydroxyethyl starch	Shock	10-20 mL/kg/day	IV (rapid infusion)	To effect. (See Appendix H)
		16 mL/kg (D)	IV	To effect
Hydroxyurea	Primary polycythemia	30-50 mg/kg (D)	PO	3 days per week
		25-30 mg/kg (C)	PO	3 days per week
		Initial dose: 0.5 g/m^2	PO	12 x 5-7 days

DRUG	INDICATIONS	DOSE	ROUTE	FREQUENCY (HR)
continued—		Maintenance dose: 15 mg/kg	PO	24 until remission then taper to minimum effective dose
	Chronic granulocytic leukemia	20-25 mg/kg (D)	PO	12 x 4-6 weeks then reduce dosage by 50%
		0.5 g/m^2	PO	12 x 4-6 weeks then reduce dosage by 50%
Hydroxyzine hydrochloride or pamoate	Antihistamine, allergic skin disease	2.2 mg/kg (D)	PO	6-12
		5-10 mg/cat	PO	12
		1-2 mg/kg	PO	8-12
Hypertonic saline	See Sodium chloride, 7.5%			
Idarubicin hydrochloride	Anticancer	2 mg/cat	PO	3 consecutive days. Repeat every 3 weeks
Idoxuridine 0.1% solution	Ocular herpes virus infections	1 drop in each eye (C)	Topical (ophthalmic)	4-8
Idoxuridine 0.5% ointment		Apply to local lesion	Topical	4-8
Ifosfamide (see also Mesna)	Anticancer	<10 kg: 350 mg/m^2 (D)	IV	Administer during the second 30 min of a 6 hr saline infusion at 18.3 ml/kg/hr. Repeat once every 3 weeks.
		>10 kg: 375 mg/m^2 (D)	IV	Administer during the second 30 min of a 6 hr saline infusion at 18.3 ml/kg/hr. Repeat once every 3 weeks

70

DRUG	INDICATIONS	DOSE	ROUTE	FREQUENCY (HR)
continued—		350-500 mg/m² (C)	IV	Administer during the second 30 min of a 6 hr saline infusion at 18.3 ml/kg/hr. Repeat once every 3 weeks
	Sarcomas	900 mg/m² (C)	IV	Administer during the second 30 min of a 6 hr saline infusion at 18.3 ml/kg/hr. Repeat once every 3 weeks
		Mesna: 20% of ifosfamide dose	IV	Prior to infusion and 2 and 5 hrs after ifosfamide infusion
Imidocarb dipropionate	*Babesiosis, ehrlichiosis*	5-7.5 mg/kg (D)	IM, SC	14-21 days
	Cytauxzoon felis	5 mg/kg	IM	14 days
	Haemobartonella	5 mg/kg	IM	14 days
Imidocloprid	Susceptible ectoparasites	10-25 mg/kg (D) (fleas, lice)	Topical	Monthly
		10 mg/kg (C)	Topical	Monthly
Imidocloprid/moxidectin	Roundworms, hookwoorms, whipworms	10 mg/kg imidocloprid/2.5 mg/kg moxidectin (D)	Topical	Monthly
	Heartworm prophylaxis	10 mg/kg imidocloprid/2.5 mg/kg moxidectin (D)	Topical	Monthly
		10 mg/kg imidocloprid/1 mg/kg m oxidectin (C)	Topical	Monthly

DRUG	INDICATIONS	DOSE	ROUTE	FREQUENCY (HR)
Imidocloprid/permethrin	Susceptible ectoparasites (fleas, lice, mites, ticks)	10-25 mg/kg imidocloprid/50-125 mg/kg permethrin (D)	Topical	Monthly
Imipenem-cilastin	*Susceptible bacterial infections	5-10 mg/kg	IM (using IM preparation), IV (slow), SC	6-8
		5-10 mg/kg (C)	IV	8
Imipramine	Narcolepsy, cataplexy	0.5-1 mg/kg (D)	PO	8
	Urethral sphincter incompetence	5-15 mg/dog	PO	12
		2.5-5 mg/cat	PO	12
	Behavioral disorder, separation anxiety	2.2-4.4 mg/kg (D)	PO	12-24
Inamrinone	Low-output heart failure	Loading dose: 1-3 mg/kg	IV (over 2-3 min)	Once
		Followed by: 30-100 µg/kg	CRI	(See Appendix H)
Insulin, glargine	Insulin dependent diabetes mellitus	0.25 IU/kg (D)	SC	12
		Glucose >360 mg/dL: 0.5 IU/kg (C)	SC	12
		Glucose < 360 mg/dL: 0.25 IU/kg (C)	SC	12
		0.25-0.5 IU/kg (C)	SC	12
Insulin, regular	Diabetic ketoacidosis	0.2 IU/kg (D)	IM	Once
		0.1 IU/kg (D)	IM	1 x 6-10 PRN
		0.05-0.1 IU/kg (D)	CRI in 5%	Based on hourly glucose dextrose check

Drug	Indications	Dose	Route	Frequency (hr)
continued –				(See Appendix H)
		<3 kg: 1 IU	IV	Initial, then
		1 IU/animal	CRI	(See Appendix H)
		3-10 kg: 2 IU	IV	Initial, then
		1 IU/animal	IV	Hourly
		>10 kg: 0.25 IU/kg	IV	Initial, then
		0.1 IU/kg	IM, IV	Hourly
	Hyperkalemia	0.25-0.5 IU/kg (D)	IV	Once. Follow with 50% dextrose
		0.5-1 IU/kg	IV	In parenteral fluids containing 2 gm dextrose/IU of insulin
Insulin, NPH, ultralente, PZI	Insulin dependent diabetes mellitus	<15 kg: 1 IU/kg (D)	SC	24; monitor
		>15 kg: 0.5 IU/kg (D)	SC	24; monitor
		0.8-0.9 IU/kg (D)	SC	24; monitor
Insulin, ultralente, PZI	Insulin dependent diabetes mellitus	0.5-1 IU/kg (C)	SC	12-24; monitor
Interferon α2 (human recombinant)	Nonneoplastic Feline Leukemia Virus (FeLV) associated disease (low dose)	15-30 IU/cat	IM, PO, SC	24 x 7 days on and off cycles
		0.5-5 IU/kg (C)	PO, SC	24 x 7 days on and off cycles
	FeLV appetite stimulation	1 IU/cat	PO	24 x 7 days on and off cycles

DRUG	INDICATIONS	DOSE	ROUTE	FREQUENCY (HR)
continued—	Feline Infectious Peritonitis (nonexudative)	30 IU/cat (C)	PO	24 x 7 days on and off cycles
	Feline Infectious Peritonitis (exudative)	2000 IU/Cat	IM	24
	Ocular herpes	10 IU	PO	24
		25-50 IU/mL saline	Topical (both eyes)	4-6
	Indolent ulcers	60-100 IU	PO, SC	24
	Immunosuppression	0.22 IU/kg (D)	PO	24. Add 3 million IU to 1 L sterile saline solution. Divide into aliquots and freeze. Thaw and dilute aliquots PRN to produce a 30 IU/mL dispensing solution
Interferon bovine beta	Nonneoplastic FeLV associated disease (high dose)	10,000-1,000,000 IU/kg	PO, SC	24 x 7 day on and off cycles
	Feline Infectious Peritonitis (exudative)	20,000 IU/cat	IM	24 x 14-21 days
	Acute Feline Herpesvirus in kittens	10,000 IU/kg	SC	24 x 21 days
Interferon, feline recombinant	Immunostimulation	1 million IU/kg	SC	48; reduce to 7 d when responding
Iodide sodium, potassium	Hyperthyroidism, sporotrichosis	20 mg/kg (C) of 20% solution	PO	12-24
	Hyperthyroidism (short term)	50-100 mg/cat	PO	24

DRUG	INDICATIONS	DOSE	ROUTE	FREQUENCY (HR)
continued—	Sporotrichosis	40 mg/kg (D)	PO	8
		20 mg/kg (C)	PO	12
Iohexol	Myelography	0.25 mL/kg	Epidural	Once
Iopamidol	Myelography	0.25 mL/kg	Epidural	Once
Ipecac syrup	Emetic	1-2.5 mL/kg (D). Maximum of 15 mL	PO	Repeat once in 20 min
		3.3 mL/kg (dilute 1:1 w/ water) (D)	PO	Ad libitum for 7 days
Ipodate	Hyperthyroidism (short term)	15 mg/kg	PO	12
Ipronidazole	*Giardia*	126-378 mg/L drinking water (D)	PO	24 x 7-14 days
Iron dextran	Anemia	10-20 mg/kg (D)	IM	Once
		50 mg/cat	IM	Once after 18 days of age
Isoflurane	Anesthesia	Induction: 5%	Inhalant	To effect
		Maintenance: 1.5%-2.5%	Inhalant	To effect
Isometheptene	Urethral antispasmodic	0.5-1 mL/dog	IM	8-12
		1 tablet/dog	PO	12
		0.25-0.50 mL/cat	IM	12
		0.5 tablet/cat	PO	12
Isoniazid	Tuberculosis	10-20 mg/kg	PO	24
Isopropamide iodide	Sinus bradycardia, SA or	0.2-0.4 mg/kg	PO	8-12

DRUG	INDICATIONS	DOSE	ROUTE	FREQUENCY (HR)
continued —	AV block			
	Antidiarrheal	0.2-1 mg/kg	PO	12
Isopropamide/ prochlorperazine	Antiemetic, antidiarrheal	0.14-0.22 mg/kg (D)	SC	12
		0.5-0.8 mg/kg (C)	IM, SC	12
Isoproterenol	Bradycardia, AV block, cardiac arrest	0.04-0.08 μg/kg	CRI	(See Appendix H)
		0.4 mg in 250 mL 5% D/W	IV (slowly)	To effect
	Bronchodilation	0.2 mg in 100 mL 5% D/W	IV	To effect at 8 hrs
		0.004-0.006 mg/cat	IM	30 min PRN
		0.44 mg/kg (C)	PO	6-12
		0.5 mL of 1:200 dilution	Inhalant	4
Isosorbide dinitrate	Vasodilator	2.5-5 mg/animal	PO	12
Isosorbide mononitrate	Vasodilator	5 mg/dog	PO	12
Isotretinoin	Feline acne	5 mg/kg	PO	24
	Sebaceous adenitis	1 mg/kg (D)	PO	12 x 15 days
	Schnauzer comedone	1-3 mg/kg	PO	12-24
	Epitheliotrophic lymphoma	10 mg/cat	PO	24
Isoxsuprine	Raynaud-like syndrome	1 mg/kg	PO	24
Itraconazole	Systemic mycoses or generalized dermatomycosis	5-10 mg/kg	PO	12-24

DRUG	INDICATIONS	DOSE	ROUTE	FREQUENCY (HR)
Ivermectin	Heartworm and hookworm prophylaxis	24 μg/kg (C)	PO	Monthly
		6 μg/kg (D)	PO	Monthly
	Microfilaricide	50-200 μg/kg	PO	Once 2 weeks following adulticide administration
	Cheyletiellosis, notoedric mange	200-400 mg/kg (C)	SC	1-2 weeks for a minimum of 4 weeks
	Sarcoptic mange, Otodectes	300 μg/kg	PO, SC	Once. Repeat in 14 days
	Demodectic mange	400-600 μg/kg	PO, SC	24 x 2-3 months. Start at 100 μg/kg and increase to higher dose. Do not administer to Collies or other working breeds unless normal P-glycoprotein is confirmed
Kanamycin	*Susceptible bacterial infections	10-20 mg/kg	IM, IV, SC	24; consider monitoring (See Appendix F)
		5-7.5 mg/kg	IM, IV, SC	12
	Gastrointestinal tract bacterial overgrowth	10-12 mg/kg	PO	8-12
Kaolin/pectin	Gastrointestinal tract protectant	3-6 g/kg	PO	2-6
Ketamine hydrochloride	Sedation	7-11 mg/kg in combination with 1.1-2.2 mg/kg xylazine	IV	To effect

IK

Drug	Indications	Dose	Route	Frequency (hr)
continued —		22 mg/kg in combination with 1.1 mg/kg xylazine	IM	To effect
		5.5-10 mg/kg in combination with 0.3-0.5 mg/kg diazepam	IV	To effect
		6.6-11 mg/kg in combination with 0.066-0.22 mg/kg midazolam IM or IV	IM	To effect
		33 mg/kg in combination with 0.22 acepromazine	IM	To effect
		16 mg/kg in combination with 0.66 mg/kg acepromazine	IM	To effect
		5.5-22 mg/kg (adjunctive sedative or tranquilizer treatment recommended) (D)	IM, IV	To effect
	Anesthesia	22-33 mg/kg (C)	IM	To effect
		2.2-4.4 mg/kg (C)	IV	To effect
	N-methyl-D-aspartate antagonist (analgesia)	0.1-1 mg/kg	IM, PO, SC	4-6
	Systemic analgesia	Analgesia, with morphine and lidocaine	CRI	(See Appendix H)
Ketamine hydrochloride/ aminopentamide/promazine	Anesthesia	0.3-0.6 mg/kg	CRI	(See Appendix H)
Ketoconazole	Systemic and cutaneous mycoses, prototheecosis, aspergillosis	10-20 mg/kg (D) 10 mg/kg (C)	PO PO	12-24 12-24

Drug	Indications	Dose	Route	Frequency (hr)
continued—	Sporotrichosis	5-10 mg/kg (C)	PO	12-24
		15 mg/kg (D)	PO	12
	Candidiasis	10 mg/kg	PO	8
	Aspergillosis, immune stimulation	10 mg/kg	PO	24
	CNS mycoses	15-20 mg/kg	PO	12
	Malassezia canis	10 mg/kg (D)	PO	24 x 30 days
		5 mg/kg (D)	PO	12
	Dermatophytosis	10 mg/kg	PO	24
	Coccidiodomycosis	10-30 mg/kg (D)	PO	24 x 3-6 months or divide dose and administer q 12 x 3-6 months
	Blastomycosis	10 mg/kg (20 mg/kg if ocular or central nervous system)	PO	12 x 2-3 months
	Histoplasmosis	10 mg/kg	PO	12-24 x 3 months
	Cryptococcosis	10 mg/kg	PO	24 (in combination with another antifungal)
	Hyperadrenocorticism	10-15 mg/kg (D)	PO	12
	To prolong cyclosporine half-life	2-7.5 mg/kg	PO	12. Monitor cyclosporine (reduce dose by 50% or more)
Ketoprofen	Antiinflammatory	0.5-1.1 mg/kg (D)	IV, PO	12-24 for maximum of 5 days
		Loading dose: 1-2 mg/kg (C)	IM, SC	Once
		Maintenance dose: 0.5-1 mg/cat	PO, SC	24

Drug	Indications	Dose	Route	Frequency (hr)
continued—	Perioperative pain	2 mg/kg	IV	Once
	Postoperative pain	1-2 mg/kg	IM, IV, SC	24 x 3 days
Ketorolac tromethamine	Analgesia	0.5 mg/kg (D)	IM, IV, PO	12 x 2 doses
		0.25 mg/kg (C)	IM, IV, PO	8-12 x 2 doses
L-Aspariginase	See Aspariginase			
L-Carnitine	See Levocarnitine			
L-Deprenyl	See Selegiline			
Lactated Ringer's solution	Maintenance fluid replacement	40-50 mL/kg/day	IV	PRN
	Shock therapy	90 mL/kg (D)	IV	PRN
		60-70 mL/kg (C)	IV	PRN
Lactitol	Stool softener, hepatic encephalopathy	250 mg	PO	12
Lactoferrin	Feline immunodeficiency virus stomatitis	40 mg/kg (C)	Topical	24
Lactulose	Stool softener, hepatic encephalopathy	0.5 mL/kg (D)	PO	8 or to achieve 2-3 soft stools per day
		5-45 mL/dog	PO	8
		2.5-5 mL/cat	PO	8
		0.25-1 mL/cat	PO	12-24
		5-10 mL/cat (diluted 1:3 with water)	Per rectum	To effect

Drug	Indications	Dose	Route	Frequency (hr)
continued−	Constipation	1 mL/4.5 kg (D)	PO	8, to effect
Lenperone	Chemical restraint	0.22-0.88 mg/kg	IM, IV	To effect
Leucovorin (folinic acid)	Methotrexate or pyrimethamine rescue	3 mg/m^2 (D)	IM, PO, IV	Within 3 h of treatment
Levallorphan	Narcotic antagonist	0.02-0.2 mg/kg	IV	PRN
Levamisole	Microfilaricide	10-11 mg/kg (D)	PO	24 x 6-12 days
		10 mg/kg (C)	PO	24 x 7 days
	Aspergillosis	2-5 mg/kg (D)	PO	48 x 5-6 treatments
		7.5 mg/kg (D)	PO	12
		0.5-2 mg/kg (D)	PO	3 x per week
	Filaroides, Aleurostrongylus	7.5 mg/kg (D)	PO	24
		25 mg/kg (C)	PO	48 x 10-14 days
		25 mg/cat	PO	48 x 3 treatments
	Hookworms	5-10 mg/kg (D)	PO	24 x 2
		20-40 mg/kg (C)	PO	48 x 5-6
	General immunostimulation	2.5-5 mg/kg	PO	Once
	Plasma cell gingivitis	25 mg/cat	PO	48 x 3 treatments
Levetiracetam	Anticonvulsant	20 mg/kg	PO	8; monitor (See Appendix F)
Levoamphetamine	Hyperkinesis	1-4 mg/kg (D)	PO	PRN
Levocarnitine	See L-Carnitine			

DRUG	INDICATIONS	DOSE	ROUTE	FREQUENCY (HR)
Levodopa	Hepatic encephalopathy	6.8 mg/kg initially, then 1.4 mg/kg	PO	6
Levorphanol tartrate	Analgesia	22 μg/kg (D)	SC	PRN
Levothyroxin	Hypothyroidism	20-32 μg/kg (D)	PO	12-24
		0.5 μg/kg	PO	24
	Myxedema coma	10-30 μg/kg (C)	PO	12
		50-100 μg/kg (C)	PO	Divide dose and administer q 12
Lidocaine	Ventricular arrhythmias	Initial dose: 2-4 mg/kg (D)	IV (slow bolus)	Administer at 10-15 min increments to a maximum of 8 mg/kg
		Followed by: 25-80 μg/kg (D)	CRI	(See Appendix H)
		Initial dose: 100 to 400 μg/kg	IV (slowly)	Once
		Followed by: 250 to 750 μg/kg	IV (slowly)	To effect
		15-50 μg/kg	CRI	(See Appendix H)
	Dental nerve block	7 mg/kg (D)	At site	Once
		2 mg/kg (C)	At site	Once
	Decreased cerebral blood flow	2.2 mg/kg	IV	Once
	Intraarticular intraoperative	0.22 ml of 2% solution, max 5 ml block	At site	Once
	Epidural analgesia	4.4 mg/kg (D)	Epidural	Once
		1-2 mg/kg (C)	Epidural	Once
		0.2 mL/kg of 2% (maximum 6 ml/dog;	Epidural	Once

DRUG	INDICATIONS	DOSE	ROUTE	FREQUENCY (HR)
continued—	preservative free; methylparaben okay) (D)			
	Analgesia with ketamine, morphine		CRI	(See Appendix H)
Lignocaine	See Lidocaine			
Lime sulfur	Sarcoptic mange	1:20 dilution (D)	Topical	Dip dog, air dry and repeat once per week x 6 weeks
		1:40 dilution	Topical	Dip dog, air dry and repeat once per week x 6 weeks
Lime water	Alkaline gastric lavage	5 mL/kg	PO	Once
Lincomycin	*Susceptible bacterial infections	22-33 mg/kg	IM, IV, PO	12-24
Linezolid	*Susceptible multidrug resistant Staphylococcus or Enterococcus	10-20 mg/kg	IV, PO	12-24
Liothyronine, T$_3$	Hyperthyroidism	4-6 μg/kg (D)	PO	8
		4.4 μg/kg	PO	8-12
Lisinopril	Afterload reduction (vasodilator)	0.25-0.50mg/kg. Maximum of 1 mg/kg	PO	24
Lithium carbonate	Cyclic neutropenia	21-26 mg/kg (D)	PO	24
		10 mg/kg (D)	PO	12
Lobaplatin	Anticancer	35 mg/m^2	IV	Once q 3 weeks

DRUG	INDICATIONS	DOSE	ROUTE	FREQUENCY (HR)
Lomustine	Anticancer, central nervous system neoplasms	60 mg/m^2 (D). Maximum of 80 mg/m^2	PO	5-8 weeks
Loperamide	Antidiarrheal, acute colitis	0.06-0.20 mg/kg (D)	PO	8-12
		0.1-0.3 mg/kg (C)	PO	12-24
		0.08-1.16 mg/kg (C)	PO	12
Loratadine	Allergic disorders, hypersensitivity	5-10 mg/dog	PO	12-24
Lorazepam	Status epilepticus	0.2 mg/kg (D)	IV, IN	PRN
Lufenuron/milbemycin	Heartworm preventative	1 tablet per appropriate sized dog	PO	Monthly
Lufenuron	Flea control	10 mg/kg (D)	PO	Monthly
		30 mg/kg (C)	PO	Monthly
	Immunomodulator	5 mg/kg (D)	PO (with food)	24
		15 mg/kg (C)	PO	24
	Coccidiodomycosis (adjuvant)	50-100 mg/kg (D)	PO	24
		15 mg/kg	PO	24
	Dermatophytosis	50-100 mg/kg	PO	Two treatments 2 weeks apart then monthly
		80-100 mg/kg (C)	PO	Two treatments 2 weeks apart then monthly
	Systemic mycoses	5 mg/kg (D), 15 mg/kg (C)		Two treatments 2 weeks apart then monthly

DRUG	INDICATIONS	DOSE	ROUTE	FREQUENCY (HR)
continued—	Nasal mites	1 mg/kg	PO	10 days x 3 treatments
Luteinizing hormone (LH)	Stimulate ovulation	50 IU/cat	IM	Once after mating
Lysine	Antiviral	500 mg/cat	PO	24 or divide dose and administer q 12 for life
Lysine-8-vasopressin	Central diabetes insipidus	1-2 sprays in each nostril	Topical	8-24
Mafenide 10%	Burns	Apply to length of 0.3-1.3 cm (0.25/0.5 inches)	Topical	12-24
Magnesium citrate	Laxative	2-4 mL/kg	PO	12-24 or to effect
Magnesium hydroxide	Antacid	5-30 mL/dog	PO	12-24
		5-10 mL/cat	PO	8-24
	Cathartic	15-50 mL/dog	PO	24 or to effect
		2-6 mL/cat	PO	24
Magnesium oxide	Antacid, laxative	1-2 mEq/kg	PO	24
Magnesium salts	Cathartic, stool softener	0.75-1 mEq/kg	IV	Over 24 hrs; constant rate infusion thereafter
		0.3-0.5 mEq/kg	IV	24
Magnesium sulfate 25%	Hypomagnesemia	5-15 mL	IM, IV over 1-2 hr	Repeat PRN (See Appendix H)
Mannitol 20%	Oliguric renal failure	0.25-0.5 g/kg of a 15-25% solution	IV (over 15-60 min)	Repeat every 4-6 hrs if necessary (See Appendix H)

M

Drug	Indications	Dose	Route	Frequency (hr)
continued –	Glaucoma	1-3 g/kg	IV (over 15-20 min)	Repeat every 4-8 hrs if necessary
	Central nervous system edema	1.5 g/kg	IV	Once
		1 g/kg of a 5-25% solution	IV	PRN to maintain urine flow
Marbofloxacin	*Susceptible bacterial infections	2.5-5.5 mg/kg	PO	24
Maropitant	Acute vomiting	1-2 mg/kg (D)	PO, SC	24
	Motion sickness	8 mg/kg (D)	PO	24 x 2 days
	Acute vomiting, motion sickness	1 mg/kg (C)	PO, SC	24
Mebendazole	Hookworms, whipworm, and roundworms	22 mg/kg	PO (with food)	24 x 3 days
Mechlorethamine hydrochloride	Lymphoreticular neoplasms	3-5 mg/m^2	IV, Intrathoracic	As part of protocol
Meclizine	Antiemetic, motion sickness	25 mg/dog	PO	24, beginning 1 hr before riding in car
		4 mg/kg	PO	24
		12.5 mg/cat	PO	24, beginning 1 hr before riding in car
Meclofenamic acid	Analgesia	1.23 mL (0.25 tsp) granules/5 kg (D)	PO	24
		1-1.1 mg/kg (D)	PO	24 x 5-7 days

M

Drug	Indications	Dose	Route	Frequency (hr)
Medetomidine hydrochloride	Chemical restraint, sedation, analgesia, muscle relaxant	0.75-1 mg/m²	IM, IV	To effect. (See Appendix H)
Medium chain triglycerides	Chylothorax	3 mL/kg	PO	With each meal
	Primary lymphangiectasis, pancreatic exocrine insufficiency	1.5-3 mL/kg Maximum of 15 mL (1 tbsp)/meal	PO (with food)	24 or divide dose and administer with each meal
		1-2.2 mL/kg/day (D)	PO (with food)	24 or divide dose and administer with each meal
	Caloric supplementation	2.5-20 mL (D)	PO (with food)	24 or divide dose and administer with each meal
		1-2 mL/kg (C)	PO (with food)	24
Medroxyprogesterone acetate	Prevent abortion	1-2 mg/kg (C)	IM	Once per week. Stop 7-10 days before parturition
	Reproductive control	2.5-5 mg	PO	7 days
		25 mg	IM	6 months
		2 mg/kg	IM	5 months
	Aggressive masculine behavior	10 mg/kg (D)	IM, SC	PRN
	Urine marking, anxiety, intraspecies aggression	10-20 mg/kg (C)	SC	PRN. Maximim of 3 injections per year
	Skin conditions	20 mg/kg (D)	IM	Once. Repeat in 3-6 months if needed
		50-100 mg (C)	SC, IM	Once. Repeat in 3-6 months if needed

M

Drug	Indications	Dose	Route	Frequency (hr)
	Behavioral disorders, male	Initial dose: 100 mg/cat	IM	Once
		Followed by: 50 mg/cat	IM	30 days
	Behavioral disorders, female	Initial dose: 50 mg/cat	IM	Once
		Followed by: 25 mg/cat	IM	30 days
Megestrol acetate	Appetite stimulant	0.25-5 mg/kg (C)	PO	24 x 3-5 days then q 48 to 72 hr
	Asthma	5 mg/cat	PO	24 x 4 months then one time per week x 4 weeks
	Endocrine alopecia	2.5-5 mg/cat	PO	24 x 10 days then q 48
	Eosinophilic granulomas	0.5 mg/kg (C)	PO	24 x 7-14 days
	Eosinophilic keratitis	0.5 mg/cat	PO	24 until response then 3 times per week
	Eosinophilic ulcers	5-10 mg/cat	PO	48 x 10-14 treatments then once every other week
	Feline plasma cell gingivitis	2.5-5 mg/cat	PO	24 x 10 days then 48 x 5 treatments then PRN
	Skin conditions	5 mg/cat	PO	24 x 5 treatments then two times per week
		Induction of remission: 2.5-5 mg (C)	PO	48
		Maintenance: 2.5 mg	PO	7 days
	To prevent estrus	If behavioral estrus: 5 mg/cat	PO	Until estrus stops (3-5 days) then
		Maintenance: 2.5-5 mg/cat	PO	7 days x 10 weeks
		If diestrus: 2.5 mg	PO	24 up to 60 days

M

DRUG	INDICATIONS	DOSE	ROUTE	FREQUENCY (HR)
continued—		If anestrus: 2.5 mg	PO	24 x 18 months
	Unacceptable masculine behavior, urine marking, anxiety, intraspecies aggression	2-4 mg/kg (C)	PO	24 x 7 days. Reduce to half dose beginning on day 8
		2.5-5 mg/cat	PO	24 x 5-10 days, then once weekly
	Urethritis, feline urological syndrome	2.5-5 mg/cat	PO	24-48 x 14-21 treatments until remission then once every 1-2 weeks
	Benign prostatic hypertrophy	0.5 mg/kg (D)	PO	24 x 4-8 weeks
	Prevent estrus	During anestrus: 0.55 mg/kg (D)	PO	24 x 32 days
		During proestrus: 2.2 mg/kg (D)	PO	24 x 8 days
	Pseudocyesis	0.5 mg/kg (D)	PO	24 x 8 days
	Skin conditions	1 mg/kg (D)	PO	24
	Unacceptable masculine behavior, urine marking, anxiety, intraspecies aggression	Induction: 1.1-2.2 mg/kg (D)	PO	24 x 14 days
		Maintenance: 0.5-1.1 mg/kg (D)	PO	Once every 14 days
	Vaginal hyperplasia	2.2 mg/kg (D)	PO	24 x 7 days early in proestrus
	To prevent estrus	25 mg	IM	6 months
Meglumine antimoniate	Leishmaniasis	100 mg/kg (D)	IV, SC	24 x 3-4 weeks with allopurinol
		200 mg/kg (D)	IV, SC	48 with allopurinol

DRUG	INDICATIONS	DOSE	ROUTE	FREQUENCY (HR)
continued—		5-30 mL (D)	IM, IP, IV	48-72 hrs
Melarsomine dihydrochloride	Dirofilariasis	2.5 mg/kg (D)	IM (deep lumbar)	24 x 2 days, repeat in 4 months
Melatonin	Primary acanthosis nigricans	1-2 mg/dog	SC	24 x 3-5 days
	Alopecia X, sleep disorders	3-6 mg/kg (D)	PO	8-12
		1-4 12 mg implants	Implant	Once
		1 8 mg implant/dogs under 25 lbs	Implant	Once
		1 12 mg implant/dogs over 25 lbs	Implant	Once
		1 18 mg implant/dogs over 50 lbs	Implant	Once
	Sleep disorders	3-12 mg/cat	PO	12-24
Meloxicam	Perioperative	0.2 mg/kg (D)	IV, SC	Once, prior to surgery
		0.3 mg/kg (C)	SC	Once, prior to surgery
	Postoperative analgesia	0.1 mg/kg (D)	PO (with food in dogs <5 kg)	24
	Antiinflammatory	0.1 mg/kg (D)	PO	24
		0.1 mg/cat	PO	24
		0.05 mg/kg (C)	PO	24
Melphalan	Multiple myeloma	Loading dose: 0.1 mg/kg (D)	PO	24 x 10 days
		Followed by: 0.05-1 mg/kg	PO	24 x 2 weeks
		Then: 0.05 mg/kg	PO	48
		2-4 mg/m^2 (D)	PO	24-48
		0.05-0.10 mg/kg (D)	PO	24 x 10 days then q 48

M

Drug	Indications	Dose	Route	Frequency (hr)
continued —	Ovarian carcinoma, multiple myeloma, lymphoreticular neoplasms, osteosarcoma, mammary or pulmonary neoplasms	1.5 mg/m^2 (D)	PO	24 x 7-10 days
	Feline infectious peritonitis, chronic lymphocytic leukemia	2 mg/m^2 (C)	PO	48
Meperidine hydrochloride	Analgesia, acute pancreatitis	3-10 mg/kg (D)	IM	PRN
	Sedation	5-10 mg/kg (D)	IM, IV (slowly)	PRN
		1-5 mg/kg (C)	IM	PRN
	Preanesthetic	2.5-6.5 mg/kg (D)	IM	To effect
		2.2-5 mg/kg (C)	IM, SC	To effect
Mephenytoin	Therapy of refractory seizures	10 mg/kg (D)	PO	8
Mepivacaine	Local anesthetic	Local infiltration as needed	Local Infiltration	To effect
		0.2 mL/kg of 2%. Maximum 6 mL/ dog; preservative free; (methylparaben acceptable) (D)	Epidural	q 30 seconds until reflexes absent
2-Mercaptopropionyl glycine	Cystinuria	30-40 mg/kg (D)	PO	24
6-Mercaptopurine	Chronic myelocytic leukemia, lymphoma	50 mg/m^2	PO	24
		2 mg/kg	PO	24 as part of a protocol

M

DRUG	INDICATIONS	DOSE	ROUTE	FREQUENCY (HR)
Meropenem	*Susceptible bacterial infections	12-24 mg/kg	IV, SC	8
	Meningitis	40 mg/kg	IV	8
Mesalamine	Inflammatory bowel disease	10-20 mg/kg (D)	PO	6-8
Mesna	Hemorrhagic cystitis associated with cyclophosphamide	40% of cyclophosphamide dose	IM, IV, PO, SC	3-4 x 6 treatments at time of cyclophosphamide or ifosfamide treatment
Metaflumizone	Susceptible ectoparasites (fleas, lice)	0.81-1.6 mL of 18.53% solution (C)	Topical	Monthly
Metaflumizone with amitraz	Susceptible ectoparasites (fleas, lice, ticks)	0.7 to 6.65 mL of 14.34% metaflumizone and 14.34% amitraz (D)	Topical	Monthly
Metamucil	See Psyllium			
Metaproterenol sulfate	Bronchodilation	0.325-0.65 mg/kg	PO	4-6
Metapyrone	Hyperadrenocorticism	65 mg/kg (C)	PO	8-12
Metaraminol	Vascular support during shock	0.01-0.1 mg/kg	IV (slowly)	To effect
		10 mg in 250 mL 5% D/W	IV	To effect
Metformin	Hyperglycemia (noninsulin-dependent diabetes mellitus)	2-5 mg/kg (C)	PO	12
Methadone	Analgesia	0.5-2.2 mg/kg (D)	SC, IM, IV	3-6
		0.2-0.5 mg/kg (C)	SC, IM	3-6
		0.05-0.2 mg/kg (C)	IV	3-6

92

Drug	Indications	Dose	Route	Frequency (hr)
continued—	Preoperative	0.2-0.5 mg/kg (D)	IM, SC	Once
		0.1-0.2 mg/kg (C)	IM, SC	Once
Methazolamide	Glaucoma	1-2 mg/kg (D)	PO	8
		1-2 mg/kg (C)	PO	12
		2-5 mg/kg. Maximum dose 4-6 mg/kg	PO	8-12
Methenamine hippurate	Urinary antiseptic	500 mg/dog	PO	12
		250 mg/cat	PO	12
Methenamine mandelate		10-20 mg/kg (D)	PO	6-12
Methicillin	*Susceptible bacterial infections	20 mg/kg	IM, IV	6
Methimazole	Hyperthyroidism	Induction dose: 5 mg/cat	PO	8-12
		Followed by: 2.5-5 mg/cat	PO	8-12
		2.35 mg/kg (D)	PO	8-12
Dl-Methionine	Urinary acidifier	0.2-1 g/dog	PO	8
		0.2-1.5 g/cat. Adult cats only	PO (added to food)	24
Methocarbamol	Muscle relaxation	Initial: 44-66 mg/kg (D)	PO	8-12
		Maintenance: 20-66 mg/kg	PO	8-12
	Controlling effects of strychnine and tetanus	55-220 mg/kg. Maximum of 330 mg/kg/day	IV	Give first half of dose rapidly until relaxation occurs then continue
		Initial: 44-66 mg/kg (D)	PO	8-12

M

DRUG	INDICATIONS	DOSE	ROUTE	FREQUENCY (HR)
continued—		Followed by: 20-66 mg/kg	PO	8-12
Methohexital	Anesthesia induction	11 mg/kg of a 2.5% solution	IV	To effect
	Induction with preanesthetics	5 mg/kg	IV	To effect
Methotrexate sodium	Anticancer	2.5 mg/m²	PO	24 or 2-3 x per week
		0.3-0.5 mg/m²	IV	Weekly as part of a proto-col
	Lymphoma	5 mg/m² (D)	IM, IV, PO	On days 1 and 5 of a weekly maintenance protocol
		0.3-0.8 mg/kg (C)	IV	On day 14 with 5 mg predni-sone
		2.5-5 mg/m²	PO	24
	Carcinomas, sarcomas	10-15 mg/m² (C)	IM, IV, PO	1-3 weeks
	High dose	5-10 mg/m² (D)	IM, IV, PO	1-3 weeks
Methoxamine hydro-chloride	Vasopressor: cardiac arrest, shock	100-800 µg/kg (D)	IV (slowly)	PRN
		200-250 µg/kg	IM	To effect
		40-80 µg/kg	IV	To effect
Methoxyflurane	Anesthesia	Induction: 3%	Inhalant	To effect
		Maintenance: 0.5%-1.5%	Inhalant	To effect
Methscopolamine bromide	Antiemetic, decongestant	0.3-1 mg/kg	PO	8. Use cautiously in cats

DRUG	INDICATIONS	DOSE	ROUTE	FREQUENCY (HR)
Methylcellulose	Laxative	0.5-5 g/dog	PO	PRN
		1-1.5 g/cat	PO	PRN
Methylene blue	Methemoglobinemia	4 mg/kg of a 1% solution (D)	IV (slowly)	To effect
		1-1.5 mg/kg (C)	IV	To effect
	Staining pancreatic islet cells	3 mg/kg in 250 mL 0.9% NaCl	IV (over 30-40 min)	Once Staining maximal at 25 min
Methylphenidate	Narcolepsy	5-10 mg/dog	PO	8-12
	Hyperkinesis	2-4 mg/kg (D)	PO	PRN
	Meningitis	5-20 mg/dog	PO	12
Methylprednisolone	Antiinflammatory	0.5-2.0 mg/kg	PO	6-12
Methylprednisolone acetate	Antiinflammatory	1 mg/kg	IM, SC	14 days
		1-5.5 mg/kg (C)	IM, SC	7 days-6 months
	Eosinophilic, linear granulomas	10-40 mg/cat	IM, SC, intralesional	2 weeks x 2-6 treatments
	Pannus, episcleritis	4-12 mg/dog	Subconjunctival	Once then follow with topical therapy
Methylprednisolone sodium succinate	Spinal trauma	Loading dose: 30 mg/kg (D)	IV	Once
		Followed by: 5.4 mg/kg	CRI	24-48 (See Appendix H)
		Or followed by: 15 mg/kg	IV, SC	Once in 2 h then q 6 h x 2 days. Taper dose over 5-7 days

M

Drug	Indications	Dose	Route	Frequency (hr)
continued—	Shock	30-35 mg/kg (D)	IV	Once
4-Methylpyrazole 5%	Ethylene glycol toxicosis	Loading dose: 20 mg/kg (D)	IV	Once
		Followed by: 5 mg/kg (D)	IV	12 x 2 treatments
		Then: 5 mg/kg (D)	IV	Once (at 36 hours after initial injection)
Methyltestosterone	Galactorrhea	1-2 mg/kg (D). Maximum of 30 mg/day	PO	24 x 5-7 days
	Anabolic agent	1-2 mg/kg. Maximum of 30 mg/day	PO	24
	Testosterone-responsive dermatosis	0.5-1 mg/kg (D). Maximum of 30 mg/day	PO	48
		5-30 mg/dog	PO	24-48
		1-2.5 mg/cat	PO	48
Metoclopramide	Gastric motility disorders, antiemetic	0.2-0.5 mg/kg	IM, PO, SC	6-8
		5 to 20 μg/kg (0.005- 0.02 mg/kg)	CRI	(See Appendix H)
	Gastric reflux	0.2-0.4 mg/kg	PO	8. Administer 30 min before meals and at bedtime
	Dysautonomia	0.3 mg/kg (C)	PO	8
	Bladder contractility	0.2-0.5 mg/kg (D)	PO	8
Metoprolol	Atrial fibrillation, hypertrophic cardiomyopathy	5-50 mg/dog	PO	8
	Beta-blockade	0.5-1 mg/kg (D)	PO	8

DRUG	INDICATIONS	DOSE	ROUTE	FREQUENCY (HR)
continued—		2-15 mg/cat	PO	8
		12.5-25 mg/cat	PO	12
Metronidazole	*Susceptible anaerobic bacterial infections	10-44 mg/kg	PO	6-12
		10-50 mg/kg/day	PO	6-12
	Cholangitis	25-30 mg/kg (D)	PO	12
	Entamoeba, Trichomonas, Balantidium	10-25 mg/kg (C)	PO	12-24 x 5 days
		10-30 mg/kg (D)	PO	12-24 x 5 days
	Giardia	8-10 mg/kg (C)	PO	12 x 10 days
		10-25 mg/kg (C)	PO	24 x 5 days
		25-65 mg/kg (D)	PO	24 x 5 days
		22 mg/kg	PO	8 x 5 days
	Gastrointestinal tract bacterial overgrowth, acute colitis	10-15 mg/kg (D)	PO	8
		10 mg/kg/day (C)	PO	12-24
	Plasmacytic/lymphocytic enteritis	10 mg/kg (C)	PO	24
	Gingivitis	50 mg/kg (C)	PO	24
	Stomatitis	15 mg/kg (D)	PO	8
	Hepatic encephalopathy	7.5 mg/kg (D)	PO	12
	Hepatic lipidosis	25-30 mg/kg (C)	PO	8-12 x 2-3 weeks

M

Drug	Indications	Dose	Route	Frequency (hr)
continued —	Other	10-25 mg/kg (C). Maximum of 50 mg/kg	PO	12-24
Metronidazole benzoate	See indications for metronidazole	1.6 times the metronidazole doses	See metronidazole	See metronidazole
Mexiletine hydrochloride	Ventricular arrhythmias	4-10 mg/kg (D)	PO	8-12. Use cautiously
		5-8 mg/kg (D)	PO	8-12. Use cautiously
	Doberman Cardiomyopathy	5-8 mg/kg	PO	8 until dog responds to amiodarone
Mibolerone	Prevent estrus (dogs only)	1-11 kg: 30 µg/day (D)	PO	24
		12-22 kg: 60 µg/day (D)	PO	24
		23-45 kg: 120 µg/day (D)	PO	24
		>45 kg, and in German shepherd and German shepherd cross breeds: 180 µg/day (D)	PO	24
	Pseudocyesis	10 times above dosage or 16 µg/kg (D)	PO	24 x 5 days
	Galactorrhea	8-18 µg/kg (D)	PO	24 x 5 days
Miconazole	Dermatophytosis	Apply topically as directed	Topical	12-24
	Ocular fungal infections	Apply topically as directed	Topical	4-12 times per day
Midazolam	Preanesthetic, sedation	0.066-0.22 mg/kg	IM, IV	To effect
		0.2-0.4 mg/kg	IM, IV	To effect, with an opioid
		0.1 mg/kg (D)	IV	To effect
		0.1-0.3 mg/kg/hr (D)	CRI	(See Appendix H)

M

Drug	Indications	Dose	Route	Frequency (hr)
Mifepristone	Abortifacient	10-20 mg/kg	PO	Once
Milbemycin oxime	Heartworm, hookworm, round-worm, whipworm prophylaxis	0.5-0.99 mg/kg	PO	Monthly
	Demodicosis	0.5-2 mg/kg	PO	24 x 1 month past negative scraping
	Cheyletiellosis	2 mg/kg	PO	7 days x 3 treatments
	Scabies	2 mg/kg	PO	7 days x 3 treatments
		0.75 mg/kg	PO	24 x 30 days
	Heartworm preventative	2 mg/kg (C)	PO	Monthly
Milk thistle (silymarin)	Hepatoprotection	50-250 mg	PO	12-24
		30 mg/kg (D)	PO	24
Milrinone	Low-output heart failure	0.5-1 mg/kg (D)	PO	12 (See Appendix H)
Mineral oil	Laxative	5-30 mL (D)	PO, per rectum	12
		1-2 mL/kg (D)	PO, per rectum	12
		5-10 mL (C)	PO, per rectum	12
Minocycline	*Susceptible bacterial infections	12.5- 25 mg/kg (D)	PO	12
		5-12.5 mg/kg (D)	IV, PO	12
		12 mg/kg with streptomycin (D)	PO	12 x 14 days
	Nocardiosis (adjuvant)	5-25 mg/kg	IV, PO	12
	Brucellosis (adjuvant)	12.5 mg/kg	IV, PO	12

M

DRUG	INDICATIONS	DOSE	ROUTE	FREQUENCY (HR)
continued —		5-15 mg/kg (C)	PO	12
	Haemobartenollosis	6-11 mg/kg	PO	12
	Atypical mycobacterium	5-12.5 mg/kg (C)	IV, PO	12
Mirtazapine	Appetite stimulant	3.75 mg/cat (0.25 of a 15 mg tablet)	PO	PRN
Misoprostol	Gastric protectant	1-5 μg/kg (D)	PO	6-8
	Atopy (adjuvant)	6 μg/kg (D)	PO	8
	Pregnancy termination (adjuvant)	1-3 μg/kg (D)	IV	Once, after 30th day of gestation
Mithramycin	Hypercalcemia	0.25-0.5 μg/kg	IV	24 x 2 treatments
Mitotane (o,p'-DDD)	Pituitary-dependent hyperadrenocorticism	Initial dose: 25 mg/kg (D)	PO (with food)	24 until initiated (approximately 10 days)
		Maintenance dose: 25 mg/kg	PO	7 days
	Adrenal tumor	25-37.5 mg/kg (D)	PO	12 x 10-14 days until initiated then weekly (adjust dose based on cortisol measurements). Requires lifelong corticosteroid support
	Adrenal destruction	Initial dose: 25 mg/kg	PO	6-8 x 25-30 days
		Maintenance dose: 40-50 mg/kg (D)	PO	7 days
Mitoxantrone	Anticancer, as part of a protocol	5-6 mg/m^2 (D)	IV	q 3 weeks
		6-6.5 mg/m^2 (C)	IV	3-4 weeks x 4-6 treatments

Drug	Indications	Dose	Route	Frequency (hr)
Monensin	Coccidiosostat	0.02% (C)	PO (by weight, in food)	24
Montelukast	Chronic allergic diseases (asthma, atopy, inflammatory bowel disease)	0.5-1 mg/kg	PO	24
Morphine SO₄	Supraventricular premature beats	0.2 mg/kg (D)	IM, SC	2-12 (determine dose and interval per patient)
	Analgesia	0.5-1 mg/kg (D)	IM, SC	2-12 (determine dose and interval per patient)
		3-15 mg/kg (D)	PO	
	Preanesthetic	0.1-0.2 mg/kg (D)	SC	To effect
	Antitussive	0.1 mg/kg (D)	SC	6-12
		0.05-0.1 mg/kg (C)	IM, SC	4-6
	Cardiogenic edema	0.1 mg/kg (D)	IV	PRN to effect (also see Appendix H)
		0.25 mg (D)	SC	PRN
	Hypermotile diarrhea	0.25 mg/kg (D)	PO	4-6
	Spinal analgesia	0.3 mg/kg (D)	Epidural	Once
		0.1 mg/kg (C)	Epidural	Once
Moxidectin	Heartworm preventative	3 μg/kg (D)	PO	Monthly
		0.17 mg/kg	SC	6 months
	Endoparasites	25-300 μg/kg (D)	PO	Monthly

DRUG	INDICATIONS	DOSE	ROUTE	FREQUENCY (HR)
continued—	Demodicosis	200-400 μg/kg (D)	PO	24
	Scabies	400 μg/kg (D)	PO	72 x 3-6 weeks
Mycobacterial cell wall extract	Immunostimulation	1.5 mL	IM (deep), IV	1-3 weeks up to 4 treatments
Mycophenolate mofetil	Autoimmune, immune-suppression, myasthenia gravis	10-20 mg/kg	IV, PO	12
N-Acetylcysteine	See Acetylcysteine			
Nadolol	Beta-blockade	0.25-0.5 mg/kg	PO	12
Nafcillin	Resistant staphylococcal infections	10 mg/kg	IM, PO	6
Nalbuphine	Analgesia	0.2-0.5 mg/kg (D)	SC	8-12
		0.2-0.3 mg/kg (C)	SC	6-8
Nalbuphine hydrochloride	Analgesic	0.75-1.5 mg/kg	IV	1-6, to effect
		0.03-0.10 mg/kg (D)	IV	1-6, to effect
Nalmefene	Stereotypic behavior	1-4 mg/kg (D)	SC	8-12
Nalorphine hydrochloride	Narcotic antagonist	0.1 mg/kg (D). Maximim of 5 mg	IV	To effect, repeat PRN
		0.1 mg/kg (C). Maximum of 1 mg	IV	To effect, repeat PRN
		0.44 mg/kg	IM, IV, SC	To effect, repeat PRN
		1 mg for every 10 mg of morphine	IM, IV, SC	To effect, repeat PRN

DRUG	INDICATIONS	DOSE	ROUTE	FREQUENCY (HR)
Naloxone hydrochloride	Stereotypic behavior	20 mg	SC	12
	Shock	2 mg/kg	IV infusion	Over 1 h. Repeat hourly PRN to effect
	Opioid reversal	0.002-0.04 mg/kg	IM, IV, SC	To effect, repeat PRN
		0.04 mg/kg (D)	IM, IV, SC	To effect, repeat PRN
		0.02-0.1 mg/kg (C)	IV	To effect, repeat PRN
Naltrexone (trexan)	Test dose	0.01 mg/kg	SC	Once
	Stereotypic behavior	1 mg/kg (D)	SC	12-24
	Behavioral disorders, lick granulomas	2.2-5 mg/kg	PO	12-24
	Behavioral disorders, adjuvant	25-50 mg/cat	PO	12
Nandrolone decanoate	Anemia with chronic renal failure	1-1.5 mg/kg (D)	IM	q 7 days x 2-3 months
	Anabolic effects, appetite stimulant	5 mg/kg (D). Maximum of 200 mg/week	IM	2-3 weeks
	Bone marrow or appetite stimulant	1-3 mg/kg (D). Maximum of 200 mg per week	IM	q 7 days
		10-50 mg/cat	IM	q 7 days
Naproxen	Antiinflammatory, analgesic	1.1-2.2 mg/kg (D)	PO	48. Use high dose less frequently. Use with extreme caution

DRUG	INDICATIONS	DOSE	ROUTE	FREQUENCY (HR)
Neomycin	Gastrointestinal *Campylobacter*	22 mg/kg (D)	PO	12
	*Susceptible bacterial infections	7-10.5 mg/kg	IM, IV, SC	24. Highly nephrotoxic
	Hepatic encephalopathy, enemas	10-20 mg/kg (dilute in water)	Per rectum	6
		10-20 mg/kg	PO	12
Neostigmine	Cholinergic activity	1-2 mg/dog	IM	PRN
		5-15 mg/dog	PO	PRN
	Myasthenia gravis	<5 kg: 0.25 mg/dog	IM	6
		5-25 kg: 0.25-0.5 mg/dog	IM	6
		>25 kg: 0.5-0.75 mg/dog	IM	6
		40 μg/kg or 0.04 mg/kg (D)	SC	6-8
		40 μg/kg or 0.04 mg/kg (C)	SC	6-8
	Diagnostic aid for myasthenia gravis	40 μg/kg (D)	IM	Once
		20 μg/kg	IV	Once
	Antidote for curiform block	1-40 μg/kg (D)	IM, SC	Once, repeat PRN. Administer with atropine
Neupogen	See Filgastim			
Niacin	See nicotinamide (also known as Vitamin B³)			Niacin can be dosed as nicotinamide with fewer side effects
Niacinamide	See Nicotinamide			
Niclosamide	*Taeniases*	157 mg/kg (D)	PO	Once

DRUG	INDICATIONS	DOSE	ROUTE	FREQUENCY (HR)
Nicotinamide	Vacor toxicosis	Initial dose: 500-1000 mg	IM	Once
		Followed by: 200-300 mg (D)	IM	8
		Or followed by: 200 mg (C)	PO	24 x 2 weeks
	Immune-mediated skin diseases	<5 kg: 100 mg/dog	PO	8, with tetracycline
		5-10 kg: 250 mg/dog	PO	8, with tetracycline
		>10 kg: 500 mg/dog	PO	8, with tetracycline
	Hyperlipidemia	Initial dose: 1.5 mg/kg	PO	12
		Gradually increase to: 12.5 mg/kg	PO	12
		50 to 100 mg/cat	PO	24
Nicotinic acid	See nicotinamide (also known as Vitamin B3)			Niacin can be dosed as nicotinamide with fewer side effects
Nifedipine	Arterial vasodilator, calcium antagonist	1 mg/kg (D)	PO	12-24
	Megaesophagus	0.25-0.5 mg/kg	PO	30 min before each meal
Nifurtimox (not available in the United States)	Trypanosomiasis	2-2.5 mg/kg (D)	PO	6-8 x 3 months
		8 mg/kg	PO	24
Nikethamide	CNS depression associated with central depressant drugs	7.8-31.2 mg/kg	IM, IV, SC	PRN
Nitenpyram	Flea adulticide	1-11.5 kg: 11 mg	PO	24

N

DRUG	INDICATIONS	DOSE	ROUTE	FREQUENCY (HR)
continued—		11.5-57 kg: 57 mg	PO	24
Nitrofurantoin	*Susceptible urinary tract bacterial infections	4 mg/kg	PO	6-8
	Prophylactic dose, urinary tract infections	3-4 mg/kg	PO	24
Nitroglycerin 2% ointment	Dilatative cardiomyopathy	5-30 mm (D)	Topical	4-12
	Heart failure	0.6-5.1 cm (0.25-2 inches)/dog	Topical	6-8
		1.3 cm (0.5 inch)/2.2 kg (D)	Topical	12
		0.3-0.6 cm (0.125-0.25 inches)/cat	Topical	4-6
		4-12 mg/dog. Maximim of 15 mg	Topical	6-8
		2-4 mg (0.25 inch) (C)	Topical	12
		2.5-10 mg	Transdermal	12 on, 12 off
Nitroprusside	Vasodilator for acute congestive heart failure	0.5 µg/kg (C)	CRI	Use 50 µg/mL dilution. Start low and increase incrementally (See Appendix H)
		1-2 µg/kg (D). Maximum of 10 µg/kg	CRI	Use 50 µg/mL dilution. Start low and increase incrementally (See Appendix H)
Nitazoxanide	*Giardia*, Cryptosporidiosis	100 mg/kg	PO	12 x 3 days
Nitroscanate	Endoparasites	50 mg/kg (D)	PO	Once

DRUG	INDICATIONS	DOSE	ROUTE	FREQUENCY (HR)
Nizatidine	Gastric ulcers	5 mg/kg (D)	PO	24
	Prokinetic	2.5-5 mg/kg	PO	24
Norepinephrine bitartrate	Cardiovascular disorders	0.05-0.3 μg/kg	IV	(See Appendix H)
		2-4 mg/500 mL (4-8 μg/ml)	IV	Infuse to effect
Norfloxacin	*Susceptible urinary tract infections	22-44 mg/kg (D)	PO	12-24
		5-10 mg/kg (C)	PO	12-24
	Salmonellosis	22-44 mg/kg (D)	PO	12-24
Nortriptyline	Behavioral disorders	0.5-2 mg/kg	PO	12-24
Noscapine	Cough, nonproductive	0.5-1 mg/kg	PO	6-8
Novobiocin	*Susceptible bacterial infections	10 mg/kg	PO	8
Nystatin	Susceptible infections	7,500 Units/kg (D)	PO	8
		100,000 Units	PO	8
		50,000-150,000 Units (D)	PO	6-8
		22,000 Units/kg (D)	PO	24
Octreotide acetate	Insulinoma (adjuvant)	10-40 μg/dog	SC	8-12
Ofloxacin	*Susceptible bacterial infections	5-20 mg/kg	PO	12-24
Olsalazine	Inflammatory bowel disease	10-20 mg/kg (D)	PO	8-12

RUG	INDICATIONS	DOSE	ROUTE	FREQUENCY (HR)
Omega fatty acids	See Derm Caps			
Omeprazole	Reflux esophagitis, gastro-intestinal ulceration	0.7-2 mg/kg (D)	PO	24 x 10-14 days
		20 mg/dog	PO	24
		<5 kg: 0.25 capsule (5 mg)	PO	24
		<20 kg: 0.5 capsule (10 mg)	PO	24
		>20 kg: 1 capsule (20 mg)	PO	24
		0.5-1.5 mg/kg	PO	24
	Helicobacter (adjuvant)	0.7 mg/kg	PO	24
Ondansetron	Antiemetic	0.1-1 mg/kg	PO	12-24
		Loading dose: 0.5 mg/kg	IV	Once
		Followed by: 0.5 mg/kg	IV	1 h infusion (See Appendix H)
	Intractable vomiting	0.11-0.176 mg/kg	IV (slowly)	6-12
Opium tincture	Antidiarrheal	0.01-0.02 mg/kg	PO	12
Orbifloxacin	*Susceptible bacterial infections	2.5-7.5 mg/kg	PO	24
Orgotein	See Superoxide dismutase			
Ormetroprim	See Sulfadimethoxine/ormetoprim			
Ormetoprim/sulfa	See Sulfadimethoxine/ormetoprim			

Drug	Indications	Dose	Route	Frequency (hr)
Oseltamivir	Susceptible viral infections	2 mg/kg (D)	PO	12 x 10 days
Oxacillin	*Susceptible bacterial infections	22-40 mg/kg	IM, IV, PO	6-8
	Endocarditis, penicillinase producers	50-60 mg/kg	IM, IV, PO	6-8
Oxazepam	Appetite stimulant	2-2.5 mg (C)	PO	12
	Behavioral disorders, phobias	0.2-1 mg/kg (D)	PO	12-24
		0.2-0.5 mg/kg (C)	PO	12-24
Oxfendazole	Susceptible endoparasites	10 mg/kg (D)	PO	24
Oxtriphylline (Approximately 64% theophylline)	Bronchodilator	14 mg/kg (D)	PO	6-8
		30 mg/kg (D)	PO	12 (sustained release formulation)
	6 mg/kg (C)	PO	8-12	
		10-15 mg/kg	PO	6-8
		47 mg/kg (D). Equivalent to 30 mg/kg theophylline	PO	12
Oxybutynin	Detrusor hyperspasticity	1.25-5 mg/dog	PO	8-12
		0.2 mg/kg (D)	PO	8-12
		0.5-1.25 mg/cat	PO	8-12
Oxymetholone	Anabolic agent	1 mg/kg	PO	12-24
		0.1-1.1 mg/kg	PO	24

DRUG	INDICATIONS	DOSE	ROUTE	FREQUENCY (HR)
continued–		1-5 mg/kg	PO	24
Oxymorphone	Sedation	0.05-0.1 mg/kg (D)	IM, IV, SC	To effect
		0.1-0.2 mg/kg (D)	IM, SC	To effect
	Preanesthetic	0.1-0.4 mg/kg	IM, IV	Once, to effect in combination with acepromazine, glycopyrrolate, or atropine
	Intraoperative analgesia	0.025-0.066 mg/kg (D)	IV	PRN
	Postoperative analgesia	0.05-0.1 mg/kg (D). Maximum of 4 mg	IM, IV, SC	1-6
		0.05-0.15 mg/kg (C)	IM, IV, SC	1-6. Tranquilizer may be necessary
		0.05-0.1 mg/kg (D) if cardiovascular disease	IV, IM, SC	2-4
	Analgesia	0.1-0.4 mg/kg (C)	IV	2-4 or to effect
	Restraint/sedation	0.02-0.1 mg/kg (C)	IV, IM, SC	Once, to effect. Tranquilizer may be necessary
Oxytetracycline	*Susceptible bacterial infections	55-82.5 mg/kg	PO	8
		15-30 mg/kg	PO	8
		20 mg/kg	PO	8
	Hemobartonellosis	20-40 mg/kg	PO	8 x 3 weeks
		7-12 mg/kg	IM, IV	12
Oxytocin	Uterine prolapse (involution)	5-20 Units/dog	IM	Once, after manual reduction
		5 Units/cat	IM	Once, after manual reduction

DRUG	INDICATIONS	DOSE	ROUTE	FREQUENCY (HR)
continued—	Acute metritis	0.5-1 Units/kg	IM, IV	Repeat in 1-2 h
		1-5 Units/dog	IM, IV, SC	Repeat in 30 min
		0.5 Units/cat. Maximum of 3 Units/cat	IM, IV	May repeat in 30-60 min
	Stimulate milk letdown	Spray	Topical (intranasal)	5-10 min before nursing
	Uterine inertia	0.5-3 Units	IM, SC	May repeat in 30-60 min
		2.5-5 Units/cat	IM, CRI, SC	May repeat in 45 min (See Appendix H)
		0.25-1 Units	IM, SC	May repeat in 30-60 min
2-PAM	See Pralidoxime			
Paclitaxel	Anticancer	5 mg/kg (C)	IV	Pretreat for anaphylactoid reaction
Pamidronate	Hypercalcemia	1.3-2 mg/kg (D)	IV (in saline as a 2 h infusion)	Repeat in 2-3 weeks
	Cholecalciferol toxicosis	0.65-2 mg/kg (D)	IV (in saline as a 2 h infusion)	Administer on days 1 and 4 postintoxication
		1 mg/kg (D)	IV (in saline as a 2 h infusion)	Administer on days 1 and 4 postintoxication
	Malignant bone disease	1 mg/kg	IV (in saline as a 2 h infusion)	1 x q 4 weeks
Pancreatic enzyme	Pancreatic exocrine insufficiency	0.5-2 tsp	PO (crush pills first)	Mix with food. If cat intolerant then dose orally. Mixing 20

Drug	Indications	Dose	Route	Frequency (hr)
continued—				necessary
Pancuronium bromide	Paralytic agent for controlled anesthesia	0.1 mg/kg (D)	IV	To effect (and See Appendix H)
		0.03 mg/kg (D)	IV	To effect
		0.06-1 mg/kg (D)	IV	To effec
		Initial dose: 0.044 mg/kg	IV	Once
		Followed by: 0.11 mg/kg	IV	To effect
Paracetamol	See Acetominophen			
Paregoric	Antidiarrheal	0.05-0.06 mg/kg (5 mL of paregoric corresponds to approximately 2 mg of morphine)	PO	8-12
Paromomycin (amino-sidine)	Cryptosporidiosis	125-165 mg/kg	PO	12 x 5 days
		150 mg/kg	PO	24 x 5 days
Paroxetine	Behavioral disorders	0.125-0.25 of a 10 mg tablet	PO	24
Parvaquone	Antiprotozoal	10-30 mg/kg	IM	24
D-Penicillamine	Copper hepatopathy	10-15 mg/kg	PO (on an empty stomach)	12
		125-250 mg/dog	PO (on an empty stomach)	12
	Cystine urolithiasis	15 mg/kg (D)	PO (with food if causes nausea)	12

Drug	Indications	Dose	Route	Frequency (hr)
continued—	Lead poisoning	33-100 mg/kg (D)	PO	Divide dose and administer q 4 x 7 days. Repeat once in 7 days
Penicillin G, aqueous (K or Na)	Meningitis, bacterial endo-carditis	20,000-55,000 Units/kg	IV	4-6
	Actinomycosis, tetanus	22,000 Units/kg	IV	4-6
	Leptospirosis	40,000 Units/kg	IM, IV, SC	4-6
Penicillin G, benzathine	*Susceptible bacterial infections	50,000 Units/kg	IM	2 days
Penicillin G, phenoxy-methyl potassium	*Susceptible bacterial infections	20-30 mg/kg	PO	6-8
Penicillin G, procaine	Leptospirosis, actinomycosis	20,000-100,000 Units/kg	IM, SC	12-24
Penicillin V potassium	*Susceptible bacterial infections	10 mg/kg	PO	8
Pentamidine isethionate	Babesiosis	15 mg/kg (D)	SC	24 x 2 days
	Pneumocystis carinii	4 mg/kg (D)	IM, SC	24 x 2 weeks
	Trypanosomiasis	4 mg/kg (D)	IM	Repeat on days 14, 16, 18, 20, 22, 24, and 26
Pentazocine	Analgesia	2.2-3.3 mg/kg (C)	IM, IV, SC	Maximum of q 4. May cause unacceptable dysphoria in cats
		1.65-36 mg/kg (D)	IM, IV, SC	
Pentobarbital	Status epilepticus	5-15 mg/kg	IV	To effect (See Appendix H)

Drug	Indications	Dose	Route	Frequency (hr)
continued—	Sedation	2-4 mg/kg	IV, PO	6 or to effect
	Anesthesia	10-30 mg/kg (D)	IV	Administer first half as a bolus then remainder to effect
		25 mg/kg (C)	IV	Administer first half as a bolus then remainder to effect
Pentosan polysulfate	Antiinflammatory, osteoarthritis	3 mg/kg	IM, SC	4-7 days
		10-20 mg/kg	PO 1-2 hrs after feeding	2 x per week
	Feline lower urinary tract disease	8-16 mg/kg	PO	12
Pentoxifylline	Dermatomyositis	20-30 mg/kg (D)	PO	8-12
	Immune-mediated dermatologic diseases	10 mg/kg (D)	PO	8
	Skin disorders	400 mg/dog	PO	24-48
		10-25 mg/kg (D)	PO	8-12
		100 mg/cat	PO	8-12
Pethidine	See Mepiridine hydrochloride			
Petrolatum, white	Laxative	1-5 mL/cat	PO	24
Phenamidine isethionate	Babesiosis	7.5 mg/kg	IM, SC	24 x 2 days
		15 mg/kg	IM, SC	Once

DRUG	INDICATIONS	DOSE	ROUTE	FREQUENCY (HR)
Phenobarbital	Status epilepticus	Loading: 3-30 mg/kg (D)	IM, IV, PO	Increase by 3 mg/kg increments to effect
		3-6 mg/kg	IM, IV, PO	12-24; monitor (See Appendix F)
		Each 3 mg/kg increases plasma drug concentrations by approximately 5 μg/mL	IV, IM, PO	
	Maintenance antiseizure therapy	2-4 mg/kg	IV, PO	12; monitor (See Appendix F)
	Irritable colon syndrome	2.2 mg/kg (D)	PO	12
	Sedation	1-2 mg/kg (D)	PO	8-12
		1 mg/kg (C)	PO	12
	Behavioral disorders, psychogenic alopecia	4-8 mg/cat	PO	12
Phenoxybenzamine hydrochloride	Acute hypertension from pheochromocytoma	0.2-1.5 mg/kg (D)	PO	12
		0.5 mg/kg (C)	PO	12
		2.5 mg. Increase in 2.5 mg increments to a maximum of 10 mg	PO	12
	Detrusor areflexia	5-15 mg (D)	PO	24
		10 mg	PO	8-12
	Relaxation of urinary sphincter	0.5 mg/kg	IV	Once
		1.25-10 mg (C)	PO	12-24
		5-15 mg (D)	PO	12-24

Drug	Indications	Dose	Route	Frequency (hr)
continued—	Endotoxemia	0.25-0.5 mg/kg (D)	PO	6-8
		2.5-10 mg/cat	PO	24
		0.25 mg/kg (C)	PO	8
		5-15 mg (D)	PO	24
		2.5-30 mg (D)	PO	8
		0.5 mg/kg (C)	PO	24
		0.25 mg/kg (C)	PO	8
Phentolamine	Hypertension from pheochromocytoma	0.02-0.1 mg/kg (D)	IV	To effect (See Appendix H)
Phenylbutazone	Analgesia	10-22 mg/kg. Maximum of 800 mg/dog	PO	8 then taper to lowest effective dose
	Phlebitis	3-5 mg/kg (D)	PO	8
	Antiinflammatory, osteoarthritis	13 mg/kg (D). Maximum of 800 mg/day	PO	8 x 2 days then taper to lowest effective dose
Phenylephrine	Vasopressor	0.15 mg/kg	IV (slowly)	PRN
		0.1 mg/kg (D)	IV	15 min, to effect
		1 mg/kg (D)	IM, SC	15 min, to effect
		1-3 μg/kg	CRI	(See Appendix H)
Phenylpropanolamine hydrochloride	Urethral sphincter incompetence	6.25-50 mg/dog. Round to nearest 12.5 mg	PO	8
		1-2 mg/kg (D)	PO	8
		1.5-2 mg/kg (C)	PO	8
		12.5 mg/cat	PO	8

116

DRUG	INDICATIONS	DOSE	ROUTE	FREQUENCY (HR)
Phenylpropanolamine sustained-release tablet	Urethral sphincter incompetence	<20 kg: 0.5 tablet	PO	24
		20-45 kg: 1 tablet	PO	24
		>45 kg: 1.5 tablets	PO	24
Phenytoin	Ventricular arrhythmias	2-4 mg/kg (D). Maximum of 10 mg/kg	IV	Increase by 2 mg/kg increments to effect
		10 mg/kg (D)	IV	8
		30-50 mg/kg (D)	PO	8
		20 mg/kg (C)	PO	7 days
	Tumor-induced hypoglycemia	6 mg/kg (D)	PO	8-12
	Anticonvulsant	20-40 mg/kg (D)	PO	8
		2-3 mg/kg (C)	PO	24
Phosphate enemas	Constipation, obstipation	1-2 mL/kg (medium and large D)	Per rectum	Once. Use cautiously. Use in normal calcemic patients may cause hyocalcemia
Phosphate, sodium	Hypercalcemia	Dilute 1-3 g with water (1:1) and administer 10-20 mL	PO	8-24 until stools are soft
Phosphate, parenteral	Hypophosphatemia	0.06-0.18 mM/kg	CRI	Discontinue when serum phosphorus >2 mg/dL. (See Appendix H)
		0.01-0.03 mM/kg	CRI	Discontinue when serum

Drug	Indications	Dose	Route	Frequency (hr)
continued—				phosphorus >2 mg/dL. (See Appendix H)
Physostigmine	Muscarinic mushroom intoxication	0.5-3 mg/dog	IM	30-90 min, PRN
		0.25-0.5 mg/cat	IM	30-90 min, PRN
		0.02 mg/kg	IV (over 5 min)	12
		0.055 mg/kg (large D)	IV (over 5 min)	12
	Ivermectin toxicity	0.06 mg/kg	IV (slowly)	30-90 min, PRN
Physostigmine 0.5%	Dysautonomia	Apply 0.3 cm (0.125 inches)/cat	Topical	8
Phytomenadione (phytonadione)	See Vitamin K$_1$			
Phthalysulfathiazole	Sulfonamide antimicrobial	100 mg/kg	PO	12
Picrotoxin (use is controversial)	Ivermectin toxicity	1 mg/min	IV (over 8 min)	Once
Pilocarpine 1% ophthalmic solution	Dysautonomia	1 drop	Both eyes	6
Pimobendan	Dilated cardiomyopathy	0.1-0.3 mg/kg (D)	PO	12
Pimozide	Behavioral disorders including dyskinetic disorders	0.025-0.1 mg/kg (D)	PO	24
Piperacillin sodium	*Susceptible bacterial infections	25-50 mg/kg	IM, IV	6-12

Drug	Indications	Dose	Route	Frequency (hr)
Piperacillin/tazobactam	*Susceptible bacterial infections	25-50 mg/kg	IV	6-12
Piperazine	Roundworms	110 mg/kg	PO	Once. Repeat in 3 weeks
		44-66 mg/kg. Maximum of 150 mg for puppies	PO	Once
Pirbuterol	Bronchodilation	1-3 puffs	Metered dose inhaler	12-24
Piroxicam	Antiinflammatory, osteoarthritis	0.3 mg/kg	PO	48
	Transitional cell carcinoma	0.3 mg/kg	PO	24 (D) or 24-72 (C)
Plicamycin	See Mithramycin			
Polyethylene glycol	Colonscopic procedure	20-33 mL/kg	PO (volume may require oro or naso-gastric tube)	In fasted (18-24 h) animal, ad-minister 2 doses 4-6 h apart the day before the procedure. Follow with warm water enema prior to anesthesia
		60 mL/kg	PO (volume may require oro or naso-gastric tube)	In fasted (18-24 h) animal, ad-minister 2 doses 4-6 h apart the day before the procedure. Follow with warm water enema prior to anesthesia
	Pre-operative mechanical cleansing	60 mL/kg	PO (volume may require oro or nasogastric tube)	The evening prior to surgery

DRUG	INDICATIONS	DOSE	ROUTE	FREQUENCY (HR)
Polyethylene glycol electrolyte solution	Electrolyte replacement	25 mL/kg	PO (volume may require oro or nasogastric tube)	Once then repeat in 2-4 h
Polymyxcin	Mycobacterial infections	2 mg/kg (D)	IM	12
Polysulfated glycosaminoglycans	Osteoarthritis	3-5 mg/kg (D)	IM	2-5 days
		2 mg/kg (C)	IM	3-5 days
Ponazuril	Susceptible protozoal infections	10 mg/kg	PO	12
Potassium chloride	Potassium supplementation	0.1-0.25 mL/kg	PO	8. Dilute 1:1 with water (See Appendix H). Not to exceed 0.5 mEq/kg/hr
	Hypokalemia	0.5 mEq/kg (D)	CRI	
		Add 10-40 mEq to 500 mL of fluids (depending on serum potassium level)	IV, SC	
Potassium citrate	Calcium oxalate urolithiasis	100-150 mg/kg (D)	PO	24
		50-75 mg/kg	PO	12
Potassium gluconate	Hypokalemic polymyopathy	5-8 mEq/cat	PO	12-24
Potassium gluconate, Kaon elixer	Hypokalemic polymyopathy	2.2 mEq/100 kal of energy (D)	PO	24
Potassium gluconate, Tumil-K	Hypokalemic polymyopathy	2 mEq/4.5 kg	PO (in food)	12-24

Drug	Indications	Dose	Route	Frequency (hr)
Potassium iodide	Sporotrichosis, pythiosis	0.4 mL/kg (D)	PO	24
		30-100 mg/cat	PO	24 or divide dose and administer q 8-12 x 10-14 days
Potassium permanganate (1:2,000)	Strychnine toxicosis	5 mL/kg	PO (gastric lavage)	PRN
Potassium phosphate	See Phosphate			Also (See Appendix H)
Povidone-iodine	Burns	Apply light coating	Topical	12-24
Pralidoxime (2-PAM)	Organophosphate toxicosis (administer with atropine)	20-50 mg/kg (D) in a 5%-10% glucose solution	IM, IV (slow over 30 minutes), SC, IP	12. Repeat first dose in one hour if no or insufficient
		10-20 mg/kg	(cats or small dogs) IM, IV	response 6-12 for at least 36 h
Praziquantel	Susceptible cestodes	<2.5 kg: 17 mg (0.3 mL) (D)	PO	Once
		2.7-4.5 kg: 28.4 mg (0.5 mL) (D)	PO	Once
		4.5 kg-12 kg: 56.8 mg (1 mL) (D)	PO	Once
		>12 kg: 11 mg (1 mL)/kg (D)	PO	Once
		2.5 kg: 17 mg (0.5 tablet) (D)	PO	Once
		>2.6-7.2 kg: 34 mg (1 tablet)(D)	PO	Once
		>7.2-13.6 kg: 68 mg (2 tablets) (D)	PO	Once
		>13.6-20.5 kg: 102 mg (3 tablets) (D)	PO	Once
		>20.5-27.7 kg: 136 mg (4 tablets) (D)	PO	Once
		>27.7 kg: 170 mg (5 tablets) (D)	PO	Once

DRUG	INDICATIONS	DOSE	ROUTE	FREQUENCY (HR)
continued—		≥5 kg: 5 mg/kg	PO	Once
		5 mg/kg (C)	PO	Once
	Echiniococcus granulosa	10 mg/kg (D)	PO	Once
	Paragonimiasis	25-30 mg/kg (D)	PO	8-12 x 2 days
	Diphyllobothrium sp	7.5 mg/kg (D)	PO	Once
	Spirometra mansonoides or *Diphyllobothrium erinacei*	7.5 mg/kg (D)	PO	24 x 2 days
	Nanophyetus salminocola	10-30 mg/kg (D)	PO, SC	Once
	Platynosum, Opisthorchiidae	20-40 mg/kg (D)	PO	24 x 3-10 days
	Susceptible cestodes	<1.8 kg: 6.3 mg/kg (C)	PO	Once
		>1.8 kg: 5 mg/kg (C)	PO	Once
	Paragonimiasis	25-30 mg/kg (C)	PO	8 x 3 days
	Giardia	2 small Drontal Plus (with 22.7 pyrantel and praziquantel and 113 mg febental)	PO	24 x 5 days
Prazosin	Arterial vasodilation, functional urethral obstruction	1 mg/15 kg (D)	PO	8-12
		2 mg/kg > 15 kg (D)	PO	8-12
		1-4 mg/dog	PO	8-12
	Urethral resistance	0.25-0.5 mg/cat	PO	8
		0.03 mg/kg (C)	IV	To effect

DRUG	INDICATIONS	DOSE	ROUTE	FREQUENCY (HR)
Prednisolone/ prednisone (++)				
General	Allergy	0.5 mg/kg (D)	IM, PO	12
		1 mg/kg (C)	IM, PO	12
	"Physiologic" Dose	0.25 mg/kg	PO	24
	Angioedema, urticaria	2 mg/kg (D)	IM, PO	12
	Food allergy, parasite hyper-sensitivity	0.5 mg/kg (D)	PO	12 to 24
	Immunosuppression	2 mg/kg (D)	IM, PO	12
		3 mg/kg (C)	IM, PO	12
		2-5 mg/kg	IM, PO, SC	12 to 24
		Initial dose: 2.2-6.6 mg/kg (C)	IM, IV, PO	24
		Then taper to: 2-4 mg/kg (C)	IM, IV, PO	48
	Antiinflammatory	0.5-1 mg/kg (D)	IM, IV, PO	12-24 then taper to q 2 days
		2.2 mg/kg (C)	IM, IV, PO	12-24 then taper to q 2 days
	Chronic therapy	2-4 mg/kg	PO	48
	Shock	15-30 mg/kg (D)	IV	Repeat in 1, 3, 6, or 10 h
Gastrointestinal	Eosinophilic ulcers, plasma cell gingivitis	1-2.2 mg/kg (D)	PO	24 x 7 days then taper to q 48
		1-2 mg/kg (C)	PO	24
		0.5-1.5 mg/kg	PO	12-24. Taper over 3 months
	Eosinophillic gastritis, enteritis, colitis	1-3 mg/kg (D)	PO	24 then taper to q 48

DRUG	INDICATIONS	DOSE	ROUTE	FREQUENCY (HR)
continued—	Plasmacytic/lymphocytic enteritis	1-2 mg/kg	PO	12 then taper dose weekly
	Lymphocytic cholangitis, chronic active hepatitis, copper hepatopathy	0.25-2 mg/kg (D)	PO	12
Central and Peripheral Nervous System	Hydrocephalus, acquired tremors	0.5 mg/kg (D)	PO	48
	Cerebral edema from brain tumors	0.5-1 mg/kg (D)	PO	24-48
	Idiopathic or immune-mediated meningitis, recticulosis, granulogoencephalitis	1-2 mg/kg (D)	PO	12-24
	Intervertebral disk disease, meningoence phalitis cauda equina syndrome spondylopathy	Initial dose: 0.5 mg/kg (D)	PO	12 x 3 days
		Followed by: 0.5 mg/kg (D)	PO	24 x 3-5 days
	Myasthenia gravis	0.5 mg/kg (D)	PO	12 initially. Slowly increase to q 24 until remission then q 48
		2 mg/kg (D)	PO	12-24
Respiratory	Allergic bronchitis and rhinitis, asthma	0.5-2 mg/kg (D)	IM, PO	12
	Chronic bronchitis	0.1-0.5 mg/kg (D)	PO	12
	Pulmonary eosinophilic infiltrates	0.5-1 mg/kg	PO	24
	Heartworm disease including	0.5-1 mg/kg	PO	12, taper over 14 days

124

DRUG	INDICATIONS	DOSE	ROUTE	FREQUENCY (HR)
continued—	hemoptysis, coughing, or pneumonitis			Prednis(ol)one may increase heartworm resistance to treatment
Hematologic	Immune hemolytic anemia	0.5-2 mg/kg (D)	PO	12
	Immune thrombocytopenia	0.5-1.5 mg/kg (D)	PO	12
Dermatologic	Immune skin diseases	1.1-2.2 mg/kg	PO	12
	Systemic lupus erythematosus	1.5-2 mg/kg	PO	12-24 then taper to <1 mg/kg q 48
	Canine atopy, contact allergy, flea allergy, acanthosis nigricans	0.5 mg/kg (D)	PO	12 x 5-10 days then taper
	Sterile pyogranulomas	2-4 mg/kg (D)	PO	24
	Juvenile cellulitis	2.2 mg/kg (D)	PO	24
Musculoskeletal	Panosteitis, hypertrophic osteopathy	0.5 mg/kg (D)	PO	12-24
	Immune polymyositis, masticatory myositis	2 mg/kg	IM, PO	24
Cancer	Lymphoma	Initial dose: 40 mg/m^2 (D)	PO	24 x 1 week
		Followed by: 20 mg/m^2 (D)	PO	48
	Lymphosarcoma, myeloproliferative disorders, eosinophillic leukemia	1 mg/kg	PO	24 then q 48 as part of a protocol
		30-40 mg/m^2	PO	24 then q 48
		30-40 mg/m^2 (D)	PO	24 x 4 weeks then every

DRUG	INDICATIONS	DOSE	ROUTE	FREQUENCY (HR)
continued—		40 mg/m^2 (C)	PO	24 x 4 weeks then every other 48
	Multiple myeloma, macroglo-bulinemia	0.5 mg/kg (D)	PO	24 as part of a protocol
	Brain tumor	0.5-1 mg/kg	PO	24-48
Urogenital	Urethritis, persistent hematuria	2.5-5 mg/cat	PO	24-48
	Immune-mediated orchitis	1-2 mg/kg (D)	PO	24
Metabolic	Hypoadrenocorticism	0.2-0.4 mg/kg (D)	PO	24-48
		1 mg/kg (C)	IM, PO	12
	Hypoglycemia	0.25-3 mg/kg	PO	12
	Hyperinsulinism	0.25 mg/kg	PO	12
	Replacement therapy (hypo-adrenocorticism) acute	Initial dose: 4-20 mg/kg	IV (over 2-4 min)	Once
		Followed by: 0.2-0.4 mg/kg	PO	24
	Adrenal gland removal (replacement therapy)	102 mg/kg	IV	At induction
	Hypercalcemia	1-2.5 mg/kg (D)	PO	12
Ocular	Blepharitis, episcleritis, uveitis	0.5-2 mg/kg	PO	12
Other	Feline infectious peritonitis	4 mg/kg	PO	24 (with cyclophosphamide)
Prednisolone acetate	Hypoadrenocorticism	0.1-0.2 mg/kg	IM	12
Prednisolone sodium phosphate	Shock	11 mg/kg	IV	Repeat in 4-6 hrs

Drug	Indications	Dose	Route	Frequency (hr)
Prednisolone sodium succinate	Chronic allergic diseases (asthma, atopy, IBD)	2-4 mg/kg (D)	IV, IM	Repeat in 4-6 hrs
		1-3 mg/kg (C)	IV, IM	Repeat in 4-6 hrs
	Shock	11-30 mg/kg (D)	IV	Repeat in 4-6 hrs
	Hypoglycemia	1-2 mg/kg	IV	Repeat in 4-6 hrs
	CNS trauma	Initial dose: 15-30 mg/kg	IV	Once
		Maintenance dose: 1-2 mg/kg	IV	12
Pregabalin	Chronic pain, anticonvulsant	4 mg/kg (D)	PO	8
Primaquine phosphate	Hepatozoosis, babesiosis	0.3 mg/kg active base	PO	24 x 14 days
	Babesiosis	0.5 mg/kg (C)	IM, PO	Once
Primidone	Anticonvulsant	Loading dose: 55 mg/kg (D)	PO	Once. Efficacy of primidone reflects metabolism to phenobarbital; monitor (See Appendix F)
		Maintenance dose: 10-15 mg/kg (D)	PO	8 to 12
		11-22 mg/kg (C)	PO	8. Not effectively converted to phenobarbital in cats
		20 mg/kg (C)	PO	12
Procainamide	Ventricular arrhythmias	25-50 μg/kg/min (D)	CRI	(See Appendix H). 500-1,000 mg in 500 mL 5% D/W, to effect

DRUG	INDICATIONS	DOSE	ROUTE	FREQUENCY (HR)
continued—		Initial dose: 6-8 mg/kg (D). Maximum of 15 mg/kg	IV (over 5 min)	Once
		Followed by: 25-40 µg/kg (D)	CRI	(See Appendix H)
		6-20 mg/kg (D)	IM	4-6
		8-23 mg/kg (D)	PO	6-8; monitor (See Appendix F)
		6.6-22 mg/kg	PO	4 or up to q 8 if sustained-release formulation; monitor (See Appendix F)
		62.5 mg/cat	PO	6; monitor (See Appendix F)
		Initial dose: 1-2 mg/kg (C)	IV	Once
		Followed by: 10-20 µg/kg (C)	CRI	(See Appendix H)
		3-8 mg/kg (C)	IM, PO	6-8; monitor (See Appendix F)
		20 mg/kg (D)	PO (sustained-release formulation)	8; monitor (See Appendix F)
Prochlorperazine	Antiemetic	1 mg/kg (D)	PO	12
		0.13-0.5 mg/kg (D)	IM	6-8
		0.1 mg/kg	IM	6
		0.13 mg/kg (C)	IM	12
		0.5 mg/kg (C)	PO	6-8
Procarbazine hydrochloride	Anticancer	50 mg/m²	PO	24 on days 1-14 as part of a protocol
	Granulamatous meningioencephalitis	25-50 mg/m² (D)	PO	24

Drug	Indications	Dose	Route	Frequency (hr)
Prochlorperazine/iso-propamide	See Isopropamide/prochlorperazine			
Promazine hydrochloride	Preanesthetic	2.2-6.6 mg/kg (D)	IV	Once
	Sedative	2.2-4.4 mg/kg	IM	4-6
	Antiemetic	1-2 mg/kg	IM, IV	4-6
	Other	2-4 mg/kg	IM, IV	4-6
Promethazine hydrochloride	Antihistamine, antiemetic	0.2-0.4 mg/kg. Maximum of 1 mg/kg	IM, IV, PO	6-8
Propantheline bromide	Sinus bradycardia	0.25-1 mg/kg (D)	PO	8
		7-30 mg/dog	PO	8
		0.8-1.6 mg/kg (C)	PO	8
		7.5 mg/cat	PO	8
	Acute colitis, irritable colon syndrome, antiemetic	0.22-0.5 mg/kg	PO	8. Maximum of 3 days
	Detrusor hyperspasticity, urge incontinence	0.2 mg/kg	PO	6-8
		7.5-30 mg/dog depending on size	PO	8
		5-7.5 mg/cat	PO	24-72. Maximum of q 8
		0.25-0.5 mg/kg (C)	PO	12-24
	Antiemetic, antidiarrheal	0.25 mg/kg	PO	8
Propiomazine	See Propiopromazine			

DRUG	INDICATIONS	DOSE	ROUTE	FREQUENCY (HR)
Propionibacterium acnes	Immunostimulation	<7 kg: 0.1-0.2 mg/dog	IV	4 x per week in first week, 2 x per week at 3-4 day intervals followed by 1 x per week until clinical signs abate or stabilize. Maintenance dose once per month.
		6.8-20 kg: 0.2-0.4 mg/dog	IV	4 x per week in first week, 2 x per week at 3-4 day intervals followed by 1 x per week until clinical signs abate or stabilize. Maintenance dose once per month.
		20-34 kg: 0.4-0.6 mg/dog	IV	4 x per week in first week, 2 x per week at 3-4 day intervals followed by 1 x per week until clinical signs abate or stabilize. Maintenance dose once per month.
		>34 kg: 0.6-0.8 mg/dog	IV	4 x per week in first week, 2 x per week at 3-4 day intervals followed by 1 x per week until clinical signs abate or stabilize. Maintenance dose once per month.

DRUG	INDICATIONS	DOSE	ROUTE	FREQUENCY (HR)
continued—	Canine pyoderma	0.03-0.07 mg/kg (D)	IV	2 x per week x 10 weeks
	Feline retrovirus infections	15 µg/kg	IV	Biweekly for 2-3 weeks
Propiopromazine	Sedation	1.1-4.4 mg/kg	IM, IV	12-24
Propofol	Anesthesia	Induction: 6-8 mg/kg	IV	To effect
		Induction: 2.5-4 mg/kg	IV	With premedication
		Maintenance: 0.51 mg/kg (C)	CRI	(See Appendix H)
		0.4 mg/kg (D)	CRI	(See Appendix H)
	Refractory status epilepticus	0.1-0.6 mg/kg	CRI	(See Appendix H)
Propranolol	Ventricular hypertrophy, aortic stenosis	0.125-0.25 mg/kg (D)	PO	12
		0.2-1 mg/kg (D)	PO	8
		0.4-1.2 mg/kg (C)	PO	8-12
	Ventricular arrhythmias	0.02-0.06 mg/kg	IV (over 2-3 min)	8 or to effect
		0.44-1.1 mg/kg (D)	PO	8
		Initial dose: 0.25-0.5 mg/cat	IV (slowly)	Once
		Followed by: 2.5-5 mg/cat	PO	8
	Hypertrophic cardiomyopathy, valvular insufficiency	0.3-1 mg/kg (D). Maximum of 120 mg/day	PO	8
		≤5 kg: 2.5 mg/cat	PO	8-12
		>5 kg: 5 mg/cat	PO	8-12

DRUG	INDICATIONS	DOSE	ROUTE	FREQUENCY (HR)
continued—	Hypertension	2.5-10 mg/dog	PO	8-12
		2.5-5 mg/cat	PO	8-12
Propranolol	Tachyarrhythmias from endocrinopathies	0.15-0.5 mg/kg (D)	PO	8
		0.3-1 mg/kg (D)	IV	8-12 or to effect
		2.5-5 mg (C)	PO	8-12
Propylthiouracil (PTU)	Hyperthyroidism	10 mg/kg (C)	PO	8
		50 mg/cat	PO	8-12
		11 mg/kg	PO	12
		150 mg/dog	PO	24
Prostaglandin F2 alpha	Pyometritis, open cystic endometrial hyperplasia	0.1-0.5 mg/kg (D)	SC	24 x 5-7 days
		0.1-0.25 mg/kg (C)	SC	24 x 3-5 days
	Abortifacient	25-60 μg/kg (D)	IM	12 at mid- to end gestation
		0.5-1.0 mg/kg (C)	SC	24 x 2 treatments at 40 days postconception
Protamine sulfate	Heparin antagonist	1-1.5 mg for every 100 IU heparin to be antagonized; no more than 50 mg each 10 min	IV (over 10 min)	Then decrease dose by 50% each hour from time of heparin administration
Protopam chloride	See Pralidoxime			
Protriptyline	Narcolepsy	5-10 mg/dog	PO	24 at bedtime

DRUG	INDICATIONS	DOSE	ROUTE	FREQUENCY (HR)
Prucalopride	Colonic motility	0.02-1.25 mg/kg (D)	IV, PO	Frequency not established
		0.64 mg/kg (C)	IV, PO	Frequency not established
Pseudoephedrine	Nasal decongestant	15-30 mg	PO	8-12
	Urinary incontinence	0.2-0.4 mg/kg or 15-60 mg	PO	8-12
Psyllium	Bulk laxative	2-10 g/dog	PO (with food)	12-24 or PRN
		2-4 g/cat	PO (with food)	8-24
Pyrantel pamoate	Susceptible ectoparasites (roundworms and hookworms)	5 mg/kg (1 mL/10 kg) (D)	PO	Once. Repeat in 3 weeks
		15 mg/kg (D)	PO	Repeat in 14 days (hookworms), every other week x 3 treatments for a bitch with previous pup loss to hookworm anemia or heavy ascarid infestation in puppies
		10 mg/kg (C)	PO	Once. Repeat in 2 weeks
Pyridostigmine bromide	Myasthenia gravis	0.2-3 mg/kg (D)	PO	8-12. Administer anticholinergic first. Start at a low dose and increase PRN
		0.3-0.5 mg/kg	PO	8-12
		7.5-30 mg/dog	PO	12
		<5 kg: 45 mg/dog	PO	6

DRUG	INDICATIONS	DOSE	ROUTE	FREQUENCY (HR)
continued—		5-25 kg: 45-90 mg/dog	PO	6
		>25 kg: 90-135 mg/dog	PO	6
		0.02-0.04 mg/kg	IV	2 (See Appendix H)
	Myasthenia gravis	Initial dose: 0.25 mg/kg (C)	PO	Once
		Followed by: 1-3 mg/kg (C)	PO	8-12
	Antidote (curariform)	0.15-0.3 mg/kg	IM, IV	To effect
Pyrilamine maleate	Antihistamine	12.5-25 mg	PO	6
Pyrimethamine	Toxoplasmosis	0.25-1 mg/kg	PO	24 x 14-28 days
	Enteroepithelial cycle	2 mg/kg (C)	PO	24 x 14-28 days (x 5 days only for *Neosporum canium*)
	Neosporosis	1 mg/kg (D)	PO	24
		0.25-1 mg/kg (C)	PO	24
Quinacrine	*Giardia*	6.6 mg/kg (D)	PO	12 x 5 days
	Giardia, coccidiosis	11 mg/kg (C)	PO	24 x 5 days
Quinidine	Cardiac arrhythmias	4-8 mg/kg(C)	IM	8
		10-20 mg/kg (C)	PO	6-8
Quinidine gluconate (approximately 60% quindine base)	Cardiac arrhythmias	6-20 mg/kg (D)	IM, IV (slow), PO	6-12
	Ventricular tachycardia	6.6-22 mg/kg	IM	2-4 (or q 8-12 if sustained-release formulation)

Drug	Indications	Dose	Route	Frequency (hr)
continued—		6-20 mg/kg (D)	PO	6-8
	Conversion of rapid supraventricular tachycardia	6-11 mg/kg	IM	6
Quinidine sulfate (Approximately 83% quinidine base)	Cardiac arrhythmias	6-22 mg/kg (D)	PO	6 or q 8 if extended capsule
	Ventricular tachycardia	6-22 mg/kg	PO	2 until arrhythmia controlled then q 6-8 hr
Racemethionine	See DL Methionine			
Ranitidine hydrochloride	Esophagitis, gastric reflux	1-2 mg/kg (D)	PO	12
	Chronic gastritis, gastrointestinal tract ulceration, gastrinoma	2-4 mg/kg (D)	PO	8-12
		0.5 mg/kg	IV, PO, SC	12
	Hypergastrinemia from chronic renal failure	1-2 mg/kg, or (D)	PO	12
		0.5 mg/kg (D)	IV, SC	12
		3.5 mg/kg (C)	PO	12
		2.5 mg/kg (C)	IV	12
Retinol (vitamin A)	Nutritional supplement	625-800 IU/kg	PO	24
Ribavirin	Susceptible viral infections	11 mg/kg	IM, IV, PO	24 x 7 days

DRUG	INDICATIONS	DOSE	ROUTE	FREQUENCY (HR)
Riboflavin (vitamin B2)	Nutritional supplement	10-20 mg/day (D)	PO	24
		5-10 mg/day (C)	PO	24
	Bartonellosis (with doxycycline)	5-10 mg/kg (C)	PO	24 x 14 days
Rifampin (in combination)	*Susceptible bacterial infections and other organisms	10-20 mg/kg	PO	8-12 (D), 24 (C), combined with a second antimicrobial
Ringer's solution		40-50 mL/kg/day	IV, SC, IP	For maintenance fluid therapy
Ronidazole	Trichomoniasis	30-60 mg/kg (C)	PO	24 x 14
Ropavicaine 0.5%	Analgesia	0.2 ml/kg of 0.5% solution (D). Maximum of 6 mL/dog; preservative free; methylparaben acceptable	Epidural	Once
Roxithromycin	*Susceptible bacterial infections and other infections	15 mg/kg	PO	24
Rutin	Chylothorax, limb lymphedema	50 mg/kg	PO	8
S-adenyosyl methionine	Hepatopathy, behavioral disorders, degenerative joint disease	<5.5 kg: 90 mg	PO (on an empty stomach)	24
		5.5-11 kg: 180- 225 mg	PO (on an empty stomach)	24
		11-16 kg: 225 mg	PO (on an empty stomach)	24

RS

136

Drug	Indications	Dose	Route	Frequency (hr)
continued—		16-30 kg: 450 mg	PO (on an empty stomach)	24
		30-41 kg: 675 mg	PO (on an empty stomach)	24
		>41 kg: 900 mg	PO (on an empty stomach)	24
	Hepatitis	17-20 mg/kg	PO (on an empty stomach)	24
		200 mg/cat	PO (on an empty stomach)	24
Salbuterol	See Albuterol			
Salmeterol	Bronchodilation	1-3 puffs	Metered dose inhaler	12 to 24
Salmeterol/fluticasone	Asthma	1-3 puffs	Metered dose inhaler	See labelled instructions
Scopolamine hydrobromide	Antiemetic	0.03 mg/kg (D)	IM, SC	6
Selamectin	Parasiticide	6 mg/kg	Topical	Monthly for fleas, ticks (*Dermacentor variabilis*) and heartworm preventative Monthly for 1-2 months for *Otodectes*, Sarcoptic mange

DRUG	INDICATIONS	DOSE	ROUTE	FREQUENCY (HR)
continued—				Once for *Ancyclostoma tubaeforme*, *Tanei cati*
Selegiline	Cognitive disorders	0.5-1 mg/kg	PO	24
	Hyperadrenocorticism	1-2 mg/kg	PO	24
Selenium	Pancreatitis, acute	0.1 mg/kg	CRI	(See Appendix H)
	Other indications	2-4 µg/kg	PO	24
Senna (syrup)	Laxative	5 mL/cat	PO	24
Senna (granules)	Laxative	2.5 mL (0.5 tsp)/cat	PO (with food)	24
Sertraline	Behavioral disorders	0.5-4 mg/kg (D)	PO	24
		0.5-1 mg/kg (C)	PO	24
Sevelamer	Phosphorus binding	200 mg/cat	PO	8-12, with food
Sevoflurane	Anesthesia	Induction: 2-2.5 MAC	Inhalant	To effect
		Maintenance: 1-1.5 MAC	Inhalant	To effect
Silver nitrate solution 0.5%	Burns	Saturate wet dressings	Topical	12-24
Silver sulfadiazine	Burns	Apply light coating	Topical	12 for several days then q 24
	Otitis externa	Dilute 1:1 w/ water	Pack cleaned ears	12
Silymarin	See Milk thistle			

DRUG	INDICATIONS	DOSE	ROUTE	FREQUENCY (HR)
Simethicone	Antiflatulance	0.5-2 mg/kg	PO	6
Skin So Soft (by Avon)	Flea repellent	44 mL/3.8 L water (1.5 oz/gal water) (D)	Topical	Use as a dip q 7 days
Sodium aurothiomalate	Rheumatoid arthritis, skin disorders	0.5 mg/kg (D)	IM	7 days x 6 weeks
Sodium bicarbonate	Renal failure	10-15 mg/kg	PO	8
	Certain toxicoses	50 mg/kg (1 tsp is approximately 2 g)	PO	8-12
	Metabolic acidosis	0.3 x weight (kg) x (target bicarbonate-patient's bicarbonate)	IV (over 30 min)	To effect based on base deficit. (See Appendix H)
		0.5-1 mEq/kg (8.5% solution = 1 mEq/mL of $NaHCO_3$)	IV (over 30 min)	To effect based on base deficit
	Hyperkalemic crisis	2-3 mEq	IV (over 30 min)	To effect based on base serum potassium
	Urine alkalization	0.65-5.85 g/day	PO	To maintain a urinary pH between 7.0 and 7.5
		50 mg/kg (1 tsp is approximately 2 g)	PO	8-12
Sodium chloride	Hypoadrenocorticism	1-5 g	PO	24
	Hyponatremia: acute renal failure	1-4 g/day	PO	Divide dose and administer q 8
	Induce diuresis, urolithiasis	0.5-1 g (D)	PO	24

DRUG	INDICATIONS	DOSE	ROUTE	FREQUENCY (HR)
Sodium chloride 0.9% solution	Replacement or maintenance fluid therapy	40-50 mL/kg	IP, IV, SC	24
Sodium chloride 5%	Corneal edema, nonhealing erosions	Apply 0.3 cm (0.125 inches)	Topical	4-12
Sodium chloride 7.5%	Shock therapy	2-8 mL/kg (D)	Rapid IV infusion	Once, followed with a balanced crystalloid
		2-6 mL/kg (C)	Rapid IV infusion	Once, followed with a balanced crystalloid
Sodium iodide 20%	Sporotrichosis	0.5 mL/5 kg (C)	PO	24
	Susceptible infections	20-40 mg/kg (D)	PO	8-12 x 4-6 weeks
		20 mg/kg (C)	PO	24 x 4-6 weeks
Sodium polystyrene sulfonate	Hyperkalemia	8-15 g	PO	8
		2 g/kg in 3-4 mL H_2O/kg	PO	Divide dose and administer q 8
		15 g in 100 mL of 1% methylcellulose or glucose	Per rectum	PRN
Sodium stibogluconate; antimony	Leishmaniasis	30-50 mg/kg (D)	IV, SC	24 x 3-4 weeks
Sodium sulfate (Glauber's salt)	Cathartic	1 g/kg (D)	PO	4 x 6
		50 mg/kg of a 1.5% solution made with water (C)	PO	4 x 6

DRUG	INDICATIONS	DOSE	ROUTE	FREQUENCY (HR)
continued –		5-20 g/dog	PO	4 x 6
		2-5 g/cat	PO	4 x 6
Sodium thiopental	Anesthesia	3-15 mg/kg	IV	To effect
Sodium thiosulfate 20%	Arsenic toxicosis	40-50 mg/kg (D)	IV	8
Somatotropin	See Growth hormone			
Sorbitol	Laxative	3 mL/kg	PO	Once or to effect
Sotalol	Ventricular arrhythmias	1-3 mg/kg	PO	12
Spectinomycin	*Susceptible bacterial infections	5-12 mg/kg	IM	12
		20 mg/kg (D)	PO	12
	Toxoplasmosis	12.5-23 mg/dog or cat	PO	24
Spinosad	Fleas	30 mg/kg (D)	PO	Monthly
Spiramycin	*Susceptible bacterial periodontitis	12.5-23.4 mg/kg	PO	24 x 5-10 days
Spironolactone	Ascites	1-2 mg/kg (D). Maximum of 4 mg/kg	PO	12
	Diuretic, heart failure	2-4 mg/kg	PO	24
		1-2 mg/kg (D)	PO	12
	Primary hyperaldosteronism, hepatic insufficiency	1 mg/kg (C)	PO	12
		12.5 mg (C)	PO	24

Drug	Indications	Dose	Route	Frequency (hr)
Spironolactone/hydro-chlorothiazide	Diuretic, antihypertensive agent	2 mg/kg	PO	12-24
Stanozolol	Anabolic agent	2-10 mg/dog	PO	12
		1-2 mg/cat	PO	12
		0.5-2 mg/cat	PO	24
		10-25 mg/kg (C)	PO	7 days
	Anemia	1-4 mg/dog	PO	24
		25-50 mg/dog	IM	7 days
		1 mg/cat	PO	12
		25 mg/cat	IM	7 days
	Anemia secondary to uremia	2-10 mg/dog	PO	12
		1-4 mg/cat	PO	12
		1-2 mg/dog	PO	12
		2-4 mg/dog	PO	12
Staphlococcal phage lysate	Immune stimulant	Initial dose: 0.1-0.2 mL (D)	SC	Once
		Then increase in incremental doses to maximum of 1 mL (1.5 mL in large dogs)	SC	1-2 x per week
		Initial dose: 0.5 mL	SC	Once per week x 10-12 weeks
		Followed by: 0.5-1 mL	SC	q 1-2 weeks increasing the dosing interval to the longest that maintains clinical control

Drug	Indications	Dose	Route	Frequency (hr)
Staphylococcal A	Immune stimulant	20 μg/2.75 kg	IP	2 x per week
Streptokinase	Thrombosis, life threatening	Loading dose: 90,000 IU or 15,000-18,000 IU/kg (D)	IV (over 30 min)	Once. Use cautiously especially in cats
		Followed by 45,000 IU/hr (D)	CRI	For 7-12 h. (See Appendix H)
Streptomycin, dihydro	See Dihydrostreptomycin			
Streptozocin	Insulinoma	500 mg/m^2 in 18-20 mL/kg saline diuresis	IV slow infusion	Add drug during the fourth or fifth hour of a 7-8 hr diuresis. (See Appendix H)
Styrid caricide (styrylpyridinium chloride plus diethylcarbamazine)	Anthelmintic	6.7 mg/kg diethylcarbamazine and 5.5 mg/kg styrylpyridinium chloride	PO	24
	Heartworm, hookworm prophylaxis	No. 20: 1 tablet/10 kg (D)	PO	24
		No. 50: 1 tablet/25 kg (D)	PO	24
Succimer	Heavy metal chelation, lead poisoning	Initial dose: 10 mg/kg	PO	8 x 5 days
		Followed by: 10 mg/kg	PO	12 x 14 days
Succinylcholine	Paralytic, controlled anesthesia	0.07-0.22 mg/kg (D)	IV	To effect
		0.06-0.11 mg/kg (C)	IV	To effect
Sucralfate	Gastrointestinal tract ulceration	0.5-1 g/dog	PO	6-8; maximum efficacy will

S

DRUG	INDICATIONS	DOSE	ROUTE	FREQUENCY (HR)
continued—				occur if administered before antisecretory drugs
		0.25-0.5 g/cat	PO	8-12; maximum efficacy will occur if administered before antisecretory drugs
	Hemorrhagic pancreatits, vomiting with renal failure	0.5-1 g/dog	PO	8; maximum efficacy will occur if administered before antisecretory drugs
	Esophagitis, gastric reflux	0.5-1g, prepared as a slurry	PO	8
Sufentanil	Premedication	2 µg/kg. Maximum of 5 µg/kg	IV	To effect (See Appendix H)
Sulfadiazine	Nocardiosis	Initial dose: 220 mg/kg	PO	Once
		Followed by: 50-110 mg/kg	PO	12
	Toxoplasmosis	Loading: 50-100 mg/kg	PO	Once
		Maintenance 7.5-25 mg/kg	PO	12
		50 mg/kg	IV, PO	12
Sulfadiazine/ trimethoprim	*Susceptible bacterial infections	30 mg/kg (C)	PO, SC	12
		30 mg/kg (D)	IV, PO, SC	8-12
	Pneumocystis carinii	15 mg/kg (D)	PO	8-12 x 14 days
Sulfadimethoxine	*Susceptible bacterial infections	25-100 mg/kg	IM, IV, PO	12-24
	Coccidiosis	Loading dose: 55 mg/kg	PO	Once
		Followed by: 27.5 mg/kg	PO	12-24

Drug	Indications	Dose	Route	Frequency (hr)
Sulfadimethoxine/ ormetoprim	*Susceptible bacterial infections	27 mg/kg (D)	PO	24 x 14 days
		Loading dose: 55 mg/kg (D)	PO	Once
		Followed by: 27.5 mg/kg (D)	PO	24 for a maximum of 21 days
Sulfaguanidine	*Susceptible gastrointestinal microbes	100-200 mg/kg	PO	8 x 5 days
Sulfamethazine/sulfame- razine	Coccidiosis	Loading dose: 100 mg/kg	PO	Once
		Followed by: 50 mg/kg	PO	12
Sulfamethoxazole	*Susceptible bacterial infections	Loading dose: 100 mg/kg	PO	Once
		Followed by: 50 mg/kg	PO	12
Sulfamethoxazole/ trimethoprim	*Susceptible bacterial infections	15 mg/kg	PO	12
Sulfasalazine	Chronic colitis	10-50 mg/kg (D). Maximim of 3 g	PO	8-12. Taper by 50% when response occurs
	Cutaneous vasculitis	10 mg/kg (D)	PO	8 until remission then taper to lowest effective dose
	Lymphocytic-plasmacytic enteritis	250 mg (C)	PO	8 x 3 treatments then q 24 h
	Inflammatory bowel disease	10-20 mg/kg (C)	PO	8-12 for 10 days then 24 hr

Drug	Indications	Dose	Route	Frequency (hr)
Sulfisoxazole	*Susceptible urinary tract infections	50 mg/kg	PO	8
Sulfobromophthalein sodium (BSP)	Hepatic function testing	5 mg/kg	IV	Once. Collect serum 30 minutes after injection
Suprofen 1% ophthalmic solution	Allergic conjuntivitis	See directions	Topcial	8-12
Superoxide dismutase (orgotein)	Free radical scaventer, osteoarthritis	2.5-5 mg/dog	IM, SC	24 x 6 days then q 48 x 8 days
Tamoxifen	Antiestrogen agent, gastric reflux	1-2 mg/kg (D)	PO	12
Taurine	Dilated cardiomyopathy	500 mg/dog	PO	12
		250-500 mg/cat	PO	12
	Central retinal degeneration	250 mg/cat	PO	12-24
	Anticonvulsant (adjuvant)	5 mg/kg (D)	PO	12
		500 mg/cat	PO	12
Tegaserod	Colonic motility	0.03-0.3 mg/kg (D)	IV	12
Teicoplanin	*Susceptible bacterial infections	3-12 mg/kg (D)	IM, IV	24
Temozolomide	Anticancer	60 mg/m^2	PO	24 x 5 days then gradually increase to 100 mg/m^2 for 5 days

T-U

Drug	Indications	Dose	Route	Frequency (hr)
Tepoxalin	Antiinflammatory, osteoarthritis	Loading dose: 10-20 mg/kg (D)	PO	Once
		Followed by: 10 mg/kg (D)	PO	24
		5-10 mg/kg (C)	PO	24
Terbinafine	Dermatophytosis	30-40 mg/kg (D)	PO	24
Terbutaline	Bronchodilation	0.01 mg/kg	IM, SC	4
		0.312-0.625 mg/cat. Maximum of 1.25 mg/cat	PO	8
		1-3 puffs	Metered dose inhaler	12 to 24
	Bradyarrhythmias	2.5-5 mg/dog	PO, SC	8
		0.625 mg/cat	PO	8
Terfenadine	Antihistamine	2.5-5 mg/kg (D)	PO	12
Testosterone cypionate	Hormone-responsive incontinence	200 mg/dog	IM	Monthly
		2.2 mg/kg	IM	2-3 days
Testosterone enanthrate	Galactorrhea	1-2 mg/kg (D). Maximum of 30 mg/dog	IM	2-4 weeks
Testosterone methyl	Anabolic effects	1-2 mg/kg. Maximum of 30 mg	PO	24
Testosterone propionate	Hormone-responsive incontinence	1-2 mg/kg (D)	IM, SC	2-3 x per week
	Feline symmetrical alopecia	12.5 mg/cat	IM	2-3 x per week; administer

DRUG	INDICATIONS	DOSE	ROUTE	FREQUENCY (HR)
continued—				with estrogen
	Urinary incontinence	5-10 mg/cat	IM	2-3 x per week
	Infertility	0.1-1 mg/cat	IM	24-48 x 3-5 treatments
Tetanus toxoid	Tetanus treatment	0.2 mL (test dose)	SC	Once. Watch for anaphylaxis x 30 min
		Then give 30,000-100,000 Units/dog or 100-500 Units/kg (D). Maximum of 20,000 Units	IM, IV	Once
Tetracycline hydrochloride	*Susceptible bacterial infections	10-33 mg/kg	PO	8-12
		7 mg/kg	IM, IV	8-12
	Brucellosis, leptospirosis, borreliosis	10-20 mg/kg (D)	PO	8 x 28 days
	Gastrointestinal bacterial overgrowth, acute colitis	10-22 mg/kg (D)	PO	8-12
	Rickettsial and Lyme disease	20-22 mg/kg (D)	PO	8 x 14-21 days
		15 mg/kg (C)	PO	8 x 21 days
	Mycobacterial infections	22 mg/kg	PO	8
	Yersinia pestis	15 mg/kg (D)	PO	8
	Urinary tract infections	17 mg/kg (D)	PO	8
	Mastitis	10 mg/kg (D)	PO	8 x 21 days
	Pleurodesis	20 mg/kg in 4 mL saline/kg	Intrapleural	Once
	Facial tear staining	5-10 mg/kg or 50 mg/dog	PO	24
Tetramine	See Trientine hydrochloride			

Drug	Indications	Dose	Route	Frequency (hr)
Tetramisole	*Filaroides*	2 mg/kg (D)	SC	Once
Thenium closylate	Susceptible endoparasites	2.3-4.5 kg: 125-250 mg/dog	PO	12 x 2 doses then repeat once in 2-3 weeks
		>4.5 kg: 500 mg/dog. Maximum of 110 mg/kg	PO	12 x 2 doses then repeat once in 2-3 weeks
Theophylline	Bronchodilator	5-11 mg/kg (D)	IM, IV, PO	6-8
		4 mg/kg (C)	IM, PO	8-12
Theophylline sustained-release	Bronchodilator	20-40 mg/kg (D)	PO	12; consider monitoring (See Appendix F)
		20 mg/kg (C)	PO	24. Administer at night
Thiabendazole	Apergillosis	10-35 mg/kg (D)	PO	12 x 6 weeks
		10 mg/kg in 10-20 mL saline or water	Nasal flush	12 x 10 days
	Penicillinosis	20 mg/kg	PO	24
	Filaroides (*Oslerus*)	Initial dose: 70 mg/kg (D)	PO	12 x 2 days
		Followed by: 35 mg/kg	PO	12 x 20 days
		50 mg/kg (D)	PO	24 x 3 days then repeat in 1 month
	Strongyloides	125 mg/kg (C)	PO	24 x 3 days
		50-60 mg/kg (D)	PO	24 x 3 days
Thiacetarsamide	Heartworm adulticide	2.2 mg/kg	IV	12 x 2 days. Entire dose should be given within 36 hrs

DRUG	INDICATIONS	DOSE	ROUTE	FREQUENCY (HR)
Thiamine (vitamin B1)	Nutritional supplement	1-2 mg/cat	IM	12 until resolution of signs
		100-250 mg/cat	IM, SC	12 until regression of symptoms
		4 mg/kg	PO	24
		Initial dose: 10-20 mg/kg (C)	IM, SC	8-12 until signs abate
		Followed by: 10 mg/kg (C)	PO	24 x 21 days
		5-50 mg/dog	IM, IV, SC	12-24
		1-2 mg	IM	12-24
		2 mg/kg	PO	24
		100-250 mg	SC	12 until regression of symptoms
Thiamylal sodium	Induction of anesthesia	4% solution: 8-10 mg/kg (0.2-0.25 mL/kg). Maximun of 20 mg/kg	IV	In incremental doses to effect
		2% solution (C or small dog): 0.4-0.5 mL/kg	IV	To effect
	With narcotic premedication	4.4-6.6 mg/kg	IV	To effect
Thiethylperazine	Antiemetic	0.2-0.4 mg/kg (D)	SC	8-12
Thioguanine	Anticancer, lymphocytic and granulocytic leukemia	40 mg/m^2 (D)	PO	24 x 4-5 days then repeat monthly
		25 mg/m^2 (C)	PO	24 x 1-5 days then repeat monthly

Drug	Indications	Dose	Route	Frequency (hr)
Thiopental sodium	Induction of anesthesia	10-25 mg/kg (D)	IV	To effect, depending on duration of anesthesia
		15.4 mg/kg	IV	After tranquilization. Administer to effect
		11 mg/kg	IV	After narcotic premedication. Administer to effect
Thioridazine	Behavioral disorders, stereotypic and aggressive behavior	1.1 mg/kg (D)	PO	12
Thiotepa (triethylene thiophosphoramide)	Anticancer	0.2-0.5 mg/m^2 (D)	Intracavitary, IM, or in tumor	Weekly or q 24 x 5-10 treatments
	Bladder neoplasia	30 mg/m^2	Intravesicularly	q 3-4 weeks
Thyroid extract	Hypothyroidism	15-20 mg/kg/day	PO	24
Thyrotropin, TSH	Provocative testing	0.1 IU/kg (max 5 IU) (D)	IV	Once, after collection of baseline sample
		1 IU/kg (C)	IV	Once, after collection of baseline sample
		2.5 IU/Cat	IM	Once, after collection of baseline sample
	Acanthosis nigrans, hypothyroidism	1-2 IU/ dog	SC	24 x 5 days
L-Thyroxine, T$_4$, levothyroxine	Hypothyroidism	22 μg/kg (D) or 0.5 mg/m^2	PO	12; monitor (See Appendix F)

DRUG	INDICATIONS	DOSE	ROUTE	FREQUENCY (HR)
continued—		20-30 μg/kg	PO	24 or divide dose and administer q 12
	Platelet dysfunction	22 μg/kg (D)	PO	12-24
Ticarcillin or ticarcillin/-clavulanic acid	*Susceptible bacterial infections	40-50 mg/kg	IM, IV	6-8
		55-110 mg/kg	IM, IV	4-8
		Initial dose: 15-25 mg/kg	IV (over 15 min)	Once
		Followed by: 7.5-15 mg/kg	CRI	(See Appendix H)
Tiletamine/zolazepam	Anesthetic for surgeries lasting 30-60 min	6-13 mg/kg (D)	IM	To effect
	Diagnostic procedure	6.6-9.9 mg/kg (D)	IM	To effect
	Minor procedure	9.9-13.2 mg/kg (D). Do not exceed a total of 26.4 mg/kg when repeat dose(s) administered	IM	To effect
		9.7-11.9 mg/kg (C)	IM	To effect
	Restraint	6.6 mg/kg (C)	IM	To effect
	Anesthesia	11-15 mg/kg (C)	IM	To effect
	Castration, lacerations	10.6-12.5 mg/kg (C). Do not exceed a total of 72 mg/kg when repeat dose(s) administered	IM	To effect
	Spay, declaw	14.3-15.8 mg/kg (C)	IM	To effect
Tinidazole	*Giardia*	44 mg/kg (D)	PO	24 x 3 days
	Stomatitis	15 mg/kg (C)	PO	24
		15-25 mg/kg (D)	PO	12

152

Drug	Indications	Dose	Route	Frequency (hr)
Tiopronin	Cystine urinary calculi	30-40 mg/kg	PO	12
Tobramycin	Resistant *Pseudomonas* infections	6-8 mg/kg (D)	IM, IV, SC	24
Tocainide	Ventricular arrhythmias	17-25 mg/kg (large D)	PO	8
		30 mg/kg (small D)	PO	8
Tolazoline	Reversal for xylazine and other sedatives	4 mg/kg	IV (slowly)	To effect
Tolfenamic acid	Antiinflammatory, analgesia	4 mg/kg	IM (first dose only), PO, SC	24 x 3-5 days per week
Toltrazuril	Hepatozoonosis	5-10 mg/kg (D)	PO, SC	24 x 3-5 days
	Coccidiosis	5-20 mg/kg (D)	PO	24
Toluene	Susceptible endoparasites	267 mg/kg	PO	Repeat once in 2-4 weeks
Topiramate	Anticonvulsant	5-10 mg/kg	PO	12
Tramadol	Analgesia	1-4 mg/kg	PO	8-12
		2.5-5 mg/kg (D)	PO	4-6
		2 mg/kg (C)	PO	12
Tretinoin	Canine and feline acne, nasal hyperkeratosis	Apply locally	Topical	24

DRUG	INDICATIONS	DOSE	ROUTE	FREQUENCY (HR)
Triamcinolone	Antiinflammatory	0.25-2 mg (D)	PO	24
		0.25-0.5 mg/cat	PO	24 x 7 days
		0.11-0.22 mg/kg	IM, PO, SC	24-48
	Feline plamacytic pharyngitis, pododermatitis	2-4 mg/cat	PO	24-48
	Feline polymyopathy	0.5-1 mg/kg	PO	24
	Esophageal dilation to prevent restricture	1-2 mg	In the esophageal submucosa	Infiltrate at 4 circumferential points
Triamcinolone acetonide	Glucocorticoid effects	0.1-0.2 mg/kg	IM, SC	24
	Anticancer	1.2-1.8 mg or 1 mg for every 1 cm diameter of tumor	Intralesional	q 2 weeks
Triamcinolone ophthalmic solution	Pannus, eosinophilic keratitism, episcleritis	4-8 mg ophthalmic solution (D)	Subconjunctivally	Once; follow with topical therapy
		4 mg ophthalmic solution (C)	Subconjunctivally	Once; follow with topical therapy
Triamterene	Diuretic	1-2 mg/kg (D)	PO	12
Trientine hydrochloride	Copper hepatopathy	10-15 mg/kg	PO	12
Triethylene thiophosphoramide	See Thiotepa			
Triethylperazine	Antiemetic	0.13-0.2 mg/kg	IM	8-12

DRUG	INDICATIONS	DOSE	ROUTE	FREQUENCY (HR)
Trifluoperazine	Antipsychotic	0.03 mg/kg	IM	12
Trifluopromazine	Chemical restraint, antipsychotic	0.1-0.3 mg/kg	IM, PO	8-12
Trifluridine ophthalmic solution	Ocular herpes virus infections	1-2 drops of a 0.1% solution	Topical	3-8
Triiodothyronine, T_3	Hypothyroidism	4-6 μg/kg (D)	PO	8
		4.4 μg/kg (C)	PO	8-12
Trilostane	Hyperadrenocorticism	3-9-9.2 mg/kg	PO	24; based dose on cortisol concentrations
Trimeprazine	Antihistamine, allergic skin disease	1.0-2.0 mg/kg (D)	PO	12
		0.25-0.4 mg/kg (D)	PO	12 x 4 days, then reduce dose by 50%
		1.1-4.4 mg/kg	PO	8
Trimeprazine/ prednisolone	Pruritus	<20 kg: 2.5 mg/dog	PO	12 x 4 days then reduce dose by 50%
		>20 kg: 15 mg/dog	PO	12 x 4 days then reduce dose by 50%
	Allergy	0.7-1.1 mg/kg (of trimeprazine)	PO	24
	Antiinflammatory	First dose: 10-20/kg (D)	PO	Once
		Followed by: 10 mg/kg (D)	PO	24
		Followed by: 3 mg/kg (C)	PO	24

DRUG	INDICATIONS	DOSE	ROUTE	FREQUENCY (HR)
Trimethobenzamide	Antiemetic	3 mg/kg (D)	IM	8-12
Trimethoprim/ sulfadiazine	*Susceptible bacterial infections	15 mg/kg	PO, SC	12
	Meningitis	15 mg/kg	IV, PO	8-12
	Pneumocystis carinii	15 mg/kg (D)	PO	8-12 x 14 days
Trimetraxate glucuronate	Toxplasmosis	10 mg/kg (D)	IV	24 x 21 days
Tripelennamine	Antihistamine	1 mg/kg	IM, PO	12
Trypan blue	Babesiosis	4 mg/kg diluted in 5% D/W to make a 1%-2% solution (D)	IV (very slow)	
Tylosin	Gastrointestinal bacterial overgrowth, chronic colitis	10-80 mg/kg (D)	PO	12 (Tylosin powder = 3,000 mg/tsp)
		6.6-11 mg/kg	IM	12-24
		25 mg/cat	PO	8
	Inflammatory bowel disease	10-40 mg/kg (C)	PO	8-12
Urofollitropin	Hypogonadotropic anovulation	2 mg/cat	IM	24
		75 U	IM	24 x 7
Ursodeoxycholic acid (ursodiol)	Hepatopathy	5-15 mg/kg	PO	24 or divide dose and administer q 12
Valproic acid	Anticonvulsant	25-65 mg/kg	PO	8

T/U/V

DRUG	INDICATIONS	DOSE	ROUTE	FREQUENCY (HR)
Vanadium	Hyperglycemia (early non-insulin-dependent diabetes mellitus)	0.2 mg/kg (C)	PO (in food or water)	24
Vanadyl sulfate	Hyperglycemia (early non-insulin-dependent diabetes mellitus)	1 mg/kg	PO	24
Vancomycin	Gastrointestinal tract bacterial overgrowth	10-20 mg/kg (D)	PO	6
	*Susceptible bacterial infections	15 mg/kg	IV (over 30 min)	6
Vasopressin, aqueous	Central diabetes insipidus	10 mUnits	IM, IV	PRN
	Provocative testing	2.5 mUnits/kg of a 5 mUnit/mL solution in 5% D/W (D)	IV (over 1 hr)	Once, after collection of baseline urine (See Appendix H)
		0.5 mUnits/kg	IM	Once, after collection of baseline urine
	Vasoplegia (refractory hypotension)	1-4 mUnits/kg/min	CRI	(See Appendix H)
Vasopressin, tannate in oil	Central diabetes insipidus	2.5-5 Units	IM	24 hours-7 days
Vecuronium bromide	Paralytic agent for controlled anesthesia	Initial dose: 100 μg/kg (D)	IV	Once
		Followed by: 40 μg/kg	IV	At about 30 minute intervals to effect

Drug	Indications	Dose	Route	Frequency (hr)
continued—		10-20 μg/kg (D)	IV	To effect
		20-40 μg/kg (C)	IV	To effect
Verapamil hydrochloride	Supraventricular arrhythmias	Initial dose: 0.05-0.15 mg/kg (D) or 1 mg/kg if normal myocardial function	IV (bolus)	Once
	Supraventricular arrhythmias	Followed by: 2-10 μg/kg/min	CRI	To effect (See Appendix H)
		50 μg/kg (D)	IV (slowly)	Repeat at 5 minute intervals until total dose is 150-200 μg/kg
		25 μg/kg (C)	IV (slowly)	Repeat at 5 minute intervals until total dose is 150-200 μg/kg
		0.11-0.33 mg/kg	IV (slowly)	Repeat at 5 minute intervals until total dose is150-200 μg/kg
		1-3 mg/kg (D)	PO	6-8
		10-15 mg/kg	PO	Divide dose and administer q 8-12
		1.1-2.9 mg/kg (C)	PO	8
	Hypertension, conversion of rapid supraventricular tachycardia	1.1-4.4 mg/kg	PO	8-12
Vidarabine	Ocular herpes virus infections	Apply 0.3 cm (0.125 inches)	Topical	4-8
Vinblastine	Mast cell tumor, lymphosarcoma	1-3 mg/m^2 (D)	IV	7 days as part of a protocol
		2 mg/m^2 (C)	IV	7-14 days

DRUG	INDICATIONS	DOSE	ROUTE	FREQUENCY (HR)
Vincristine	Transmissible venereal tumor	0.025 mg/kg (D)	IV	7 days x 4-6 weeks
		0.5-0.75 mg/m² (D). Maximim of 1 mg	IV	7-14 days
		0.02 mg/kg (D)	IV	7 days
	Immune-mediated thrombocytopenia	0.01-0.025 mg/kg	IV	7-10 days
	Lymphosarcoma	0.5-1 mg/m²	IV	7 days as part of a protocol
	Neoplasia	0.5-0.75 mg/m²	IV	7-14 days
Viokase	Pancreatic exocrine insufficiency	3 x 325 mg tablets or 2.2-4.4 g (1-2 tsp) of powder (D)	PO	With each meal
		1 x 325 mg tablet or 1.1-2.2 g (0.5-1 tsp) of powder (C)	PO	With each meal
Vitamin A	Nutritional supplement	400 IU/kg	PO	24 x 10 days
	Vitamin A-responsive dermatosis	10,000 IU/dog	PO	24
Vitamin B₁	See Thiamine			
Vitamin B₂, riboflavin	Nutritional supplement	10-20 mg/dog	PO	24
		5-10 mg/cat	PO	24
Vitamin B₃	See Niacin			
Vitamin B₁₂	Nutritional supplement	100-200 μg/dog	PO, SC	24

DRUG	INDICATIONS	DOSE	ROUTE	FREQUENCY (HR)
continued–		50-100 μg/cat	PO, SC	24
	Inherited B12 malabsorption	0.25-1 mg/dog	SC, IM	7 days x 1 month then q 3 months
Vitamin B complex		0.5-2 mL/dog	IM, IV, SC	24 and (See Appendix H)
		0.5-1 mL/cat	IM, IV, SC	24
Vitamin C	See Ascorbic acid			
Vitamin D, cholecalciferol	Hypocalcemia	500-2000 Units/kg	PO	24
Vitamin D, dihydrotachysterol	Hypocalcemia	Loading dose: 0.03-0.06 mg/kg	PO	24 x 3 days
		Followed by: 0.02-0.03 mg/kg	PO	24 x 3 days
		Thereafter: 0.01-0.02 mg/kg	PO	24
	Hypocalcemia with renal disease	0.125 mg/dog	PO	3 times per week
Vitamin B2, ergocalciferol	Hypocalcemia	Initial: 4000-6000 Units/kg	PO	Once
		Maintenance 500-2000 Units/kg	PO	24
Vitamin B3, calcitriol, 1,25-Dihydroxycholecal-ciferol, 1,25-dihydroxy-vitamin D	Hypocalcemia	0.03-0.06 μg/kg (30 to 60 ng/kg)	PO	24
		1.65-3.62 ng/kg	PO	24. Monitor calcium. Do not administer if serum calcium x phosphorus >60

Drug	Indications	Dose	Route	Frequency (hr)
continued—	Idiopathic seborrhea	10 ng/kg	PO	24
Vitamin E	Scotty cramp	70 IU/kg (D)	IM	PRN
	Malabsorption syndromes	100-500 IU/dog	PO	24 x 4 week
	Discoid lupus, panniculitis	200-800 IU/dog	PO, Topical	12
	Vitamin E-deficient myositis, dermatomyositis	400 IU/dog	PO	24 or divide dose and administer q 12
	Acanthosis nigricans	200 IU/dog	PO	12
	Steatitis	10-20 IU/kg (C)	PO	12
	Immune-mediated skin disease	400-600 IU	PO	12
		100-400 IU	PO	12
		500 mg/dog	PO	24
		100 mg/cat	PO	24
Vitamin K1, phytonadione	Chronic liver disease	1-5 mg/kg	PO, SC	12. Recheck coagulation at 2 days and 3 weeks
		1 mg/kg/day	PO	24 x 4-6 weeks
		5 mg/kg (C)	IM	12-24
		Loading dose: 2.5 mg/kg (small D)	SC (several sites)	Once
		Followed by: 0.25-2.5 mg/kg	PO	Divide dose and administer q 8-12
		Loading dose: 5 mg/kg (large D)	SC (several sites)	Once
		Followed by: 5 mg/kg	PO	Divide dose and administer q 8-12

DRUG	INDICATIONS	DOSE	ROUTE	FREQUENCY (HR)
continued—	Acute hepatopathy	2-3 mg/kg (small D)	SC	12, until coagulation normal
		5 mg/kg (large D)	SC	12, until coagulation normal
		15-25 mg/small cat	IV	24 x 7 or until coagulation normal
		15-25 mg/large cat	IV	24 x 3-4 weeks until coagulation normal. Check 1-2 days after therapy discontinued
	Short-acting rodenticides (warfarin, fumarin, pindone, valone)	1 mg/kg	PO, SC	24 x 5-7 days
	Long-acting rodenticides (bromadiolone, brodifacoun, diphacinone, chlorphacinone)	3-5 mg/kg	PO, SC	24 x 4-6 weeks
Voriconazole	Aspergillosis, susceptible fungal infections	3-6 mg/kg (D)	PO	12-24. Use higher dose once daily. Dose has not been verified
Warfarin	Prevent thromboembolism	0.05-0.22 mg/kg (D)	PO	12-24 to maintain prothrombin time (PT) at 1.5 times baseline
		0.06-0.2 mg/kg (C)	PO	24 to maintain PT at 2-2.5 times baseline
Xylazine	Sedation, analgesia, muscle relaxation	1.1 mg/kg (D)	IV	To effect
		1.1-2.2 mg/kg	IM, SC	To effect

V-W-X

Drug	Indications	Dose	Route	Frequency (hr)
continued—	Hypoglycemic crisis	1.1 mg/kg (D)	IM	To effect
	Emetic	0.44 mg/kg (C)	IM	To effect
Xylocaine	See Lidocaine			
Yohimbine	Narcolepsy, xylazine reversal	50-100 μg/kg (D)	SC	8-12
		0.11 mg/kg (D)	IV	To effect
		0.25-0.5 mg/kg	IM, SC	12
		0.5 mg/kg (C)	IV	To effect
Zafirlukast	Chronic allergic disease (asthma, atopy, inflammatory bowel disease)	1-2 mg/kg	PO	12-24
		20 mg/dog	PO	24
Zidovudine	Antiviral	5-20 mg/kg (C)	PO, SC	8-12
Zinc acetate	Copper hepatotoxicosis	5-10 mg/kg (D)	PO	12
		Initial dose: 100 mg/dog	PO	12 x 3 months
		Maintenance dose: 50 mg/dog	PO	12
Zinc methionine	Zinc deficiency	1.7 mg/kg (D)	PO	24
Zinc sulfate	Zinc deficiency	10 mg/kg (D)	PO	24
	Copper hepatotoxicosis	5-10 mg/kg (D)	PO	12
Zolazepam-Tiletamine	See Tiletamine/zolazepan			
Zonisamide	Anticonvulsant	3-8 mg/kg	PO	12; monitor (See Appendix F)

XYZ

This list is intended to help the reader "match" therapeutic need with drug names. The list is not comprehensive and provides no indication of preferred drugs. It is incumbent on the user to understand the risks and benefits associated with the use of any drug or other compound used as a drug.

Antibacterial/Antiviral

Acyclovir
Amikacin
Amoxicillin
Amoxicillin/clavulanic acid
Ampicillin
Azithromycin
Aztreonam
Carbenicillin
Carbenicillin indanyl sodium
Cefaclor
Cefadroxil
Cefamandole
Cefazolin sodium
Cefepime
Cefixime hydrochloride
Cefmetazole sodium
Cefoperazone sodium
Cefotaxime sodium
Cefotetan sodium
Cefovecin
Cefoxitin sodium
Cefpodoxime proxetil
Ceftazidime
Ceftiofur
Ceftizoxime
Ceftriaxone
Cefuroxime axetil or sodium

Antibacterial/Antiviral *(continued)*

Cephalexin
Cephaloridine
Cephalothin
Cephamandole
Cephapirin
Cephradine
Chloramphenicol palmitate or sodium succinate
Chlorhexidine 0.5%
Chlortetracycline
Ciprofloxacin
Clarithromycin
Clindamycin
Clofazimine
Cloxacillin
Dicloxacillin
Difloxacin
Doxycycline
Enrofloxacin
Erythromycin
Ethambutol
Florfenicol

Fluconazole
Foscarnet sodium
Gentamicin
Hetacillin
Idarubicin hydrochloride
Idoxuridine 0.1% solution
Imipenem-cilastin
Isoniazid
Kanamycin
Lincomycin
Lysine
Mafenide 10%
Marbofloxacin
Meropenem
Methicillin
Minocycline
Nafcillin
Neomycin
Nitrofurantoin
Norfloxacin
Novobiocin

Antibacterial/Antiviral (continued)

Ofloxacin
Orbifloxacin
Ormetroprim
Oseltimavir
Oxacillin
Oxytetracycline
Penicillin G, aqueous
Penicillin G, benzathine
Penicillin G, procaine
Penicillin V, potassium
Piperacillin sodium
Piperacillin/tazobactam
Polymyxin B
Ribavirin
Rifampin
Roxithromycin
Silver sulfadiazine
Streptomycin, dihydro
Sulfadiazine
Sulfadiazine/trimethoprim
Sulfadimethoxine
Sulfadimethoxine/ormetoprim
Sulfamethoxazole
Sulfamethoxazole/trimethoprim
Sulfisoxazole
Teicoplanin
Tetracycline hydrochloride
Ticarcillin or ticarcillin/clavulanate
Tobramycin
Trimethoprim/sulfadiazine
Tylosin
Vancomycin

Antidotes/Therapies for Toxins

Acepromazine
Acetylcysteine
Activated charcoal
Amphetamine SO_4
Antivenin
Apomorphine
Ascorbic acid
Atropine
BAL

Antidotes/Therapies for Toxins *(continued)*

Calcium EDTA
Cascara sagrada
Castor oil
Charcoal, activated
Deferoxamine mesylate
Dexrazoxane
Dimercaprol (BAL)
Diphenylthiocarbazone
Edetate (EDTA) calcium disodium
Endotoxin antisera
Ethanol 20%
Ferric cyanoferrate
Fomepizole
Glyceryl guaiacolate
Glyceryl monacetate
Hydrogen peroxide 3%
Ipecac syrup
Leucovorin (folinic acid)
Lime water
Magnesium hydroxide
Mesna

Methocarbamol
4-Methylpyrazole 5%
N-Acetylcysteine
Nikethamide
D-Penicillamine
Physostigmine
Potassium permanganate (1:2000)
Pralidoxime
Protopam chloride
Sodium bicarbonate
Sodium sulfate (Glauber's salt)
Sodium thiosulfate 20%
Succimer
Tetanus toxoid
Thiamine, vitamin B$_1$
Tolazoline
Trientine hydrochloride
Xylazine
Yohimbine

Antifungal Agents

Amphotericin B
Captan powder 50%
Clotrimazole
Enilconazole
Flucytosine
Griseofulvin (microsize or ultramicrosize)
Iodide sodium, potassium
Itraconazole
Ketoconazole
Miconazole
Natamycin
Nystatin
Potassium iodide
Rifampin
Sodium iodide 20%
Thiabendazole
Voriconazole

AntiInflammatory Drugs—Antihistamines—Analgesics

Acetaminophen
Acetaminophen with codeine

Amantadine
6-Aminosalicylic acid
Aprotinin
Aspirin
Astemizole
Beclomethasone diprorionate
Budesonide
Carprofen
Cetrazine
Chlorpheniramine
Chondroitin sulfate
Clemastine
Colchicine
Cortisone acetate
Deferoxamine
Deracoxib
Dexamethasone
Dexamethasone sodium phosphate
Diphenhydramine hydrochloride
Dipyrone
Doxylamine succinate
Etodolac

AntiInflammatory Drugs—Antihistamines—Analgesics (*continued*)

Firocoxib
Flumethasone
Flunixin meglumine
Glucosamine
Gold sodium thiomalate
Hyaluronate
Hydrocortisone
Hydrocortisone sodium succinate
Hydroxyzine
Ibuprofen
Indomethacin
Ketoprofen
Ketoroiac tromethamine
Levorphanol tartrate
Loratadine
Meclofenamic acid
Meloxicam
Mepivacaine
Mesalamine
Methadone

Methylprednisolone acetate
Methylprednisolone sodium succinate
Montelukast
N-Acetylcysteine
Orgotein
Osalazine
Pentosan polysulfate
Pentoxifylline
Phenylbutazone
Piroxicam
Polysulfated glycosaminoglycans
Prednisolone acetate
Prednisolone sodium phosphate
Prednisolone sodium succinate
Pyrilamine maleate
Rutin
Selenium
Sodium aurothiomalate
Temaril-P
Terfenadine

AntiInflammatory Drugs—Antihistamines—Analgesics *(continued)*

Tolfenamic acid
Tramadol
Triamcinolone
Triamcinolone ophthalmic
Trimeprazine
Tripelennamine
Zafirlukast

Antiparasitic/Antiprotozoal Drugs

Albendazole
Amitraz
Amprolium
Antimony
Atovaquaone
Baquiloprim-sulfamethoxine
Benzimidazole
Bunamidine
Butamisole
Cythioate
Decoquinate
Dichlorvos
Diethylcarbamazine

Diminazene aceturate
Disophenol
Dithiazanine iodide
Epsiprantel
Febantel
Fenbendazole
Fenthion
Furazolidone
Imidocloprid
Imidocloprid with moxidectin
Imidocloprid with permethrin
Imidocarb dipropionate
Ipronidazole
Ivermectin
Levamisole
Lime sulfur suspension
Lufenuron
Mebendazole
Meglumine antimonate
Melarsomine hydrochloride
Metronidazole

Antiparasitic/Antiprotozoal Drugs *(continued)*

Milbemycin oxime
Moxidectin
Naproxen
Niclosamide
Nifurtimox
Nitenpyram
Nitazoxanide
Paromomycin
Parvaquone
Pentamidine isethionate
Phenamidine isethionate
Piperazine
Ponazuril
Praziquantel
Primaquine phosphate
Pyrantel pamoate
Pyrimethamine
Quinacrine
Selamectin
Skin So Soft by Avon
Sodium stibogluconate

Spinosad
Spiramycin
Styrylpyridinium DEC
Sulfadiazine/trimethoprim
Sulfadimethoxine
Sulfaguanidine
Sulfamethazine
Tetramisole
Thiabendazole
Thiacetarsamide
Tinidazole
Toltrazuril
Toluene
Trimetraxate glucuronate
Trypan blue

Behavior Modifiers

Alprazolam
Amitriptyline hydrochloride
Buspirone
Carbamazepine

Behavior Modifiers *(continued)*

Chlordiazepoxide
Clomipramine
Deprenyl
Dextroamphetamine
Diazepam
Doxepin hydrochloride
Fluoxetine
Fluvoxamine
L-Deprenyl
Levo-amphetamine
Lithium carbonate
Medroxyprogesterone acetate
Megestrol acetate
Methylphenidate
Nalmefene
Naloxone hydrochloride
Naltrexone
Nortriptyline
Paroxetine
Pimozide
Selegiline
Thioridazine

Blood or Blood-Forming Units

Damazol
Dicoumarol
Erythropoietin
Filgrastim (Granulocyte Colony-Stimulating Factor; GCSF)
Graunlocytecolony stimulating factor
Hemoglobin
Heparin
Lithium carbonate
Nandrolone decanoate
Neupogen
Oxymetholone
Pentoxifylline
Protamine sulfate
Stanozolol
Vitamin B_2 (riboflavin)
Vitamin K_1 (aquamephyton)

Cardiovascular Drugs

Acepromazine
Aldactone
Amiodarone

Cardiovascular Drugs *(continued)*

Amlodipine besylate

Amrinone

Aprindine

Atenolol

Atropine

Benazepril

Calcium Chloride 10%

Calcium gluconate 10%

Captopril

Carvedilol

Chlorothiazide

Coenzyme Q

Dalteparin

Digitoxin

Digoxin

Diltiazem

Diltiazem XR, Cardiazem CD

Disopyramide PO4

Dobutamine hydrochloride

Dopamine hydrochloride

Enalapril

Enoxaparin

Epinephrine

Esmolol

Furosemide

Glycopyrrolate

Heparin

Hydralazine

Hydrochlorothiazide

Inamarone

Isopropamide iodide

Isoproterenol

Isosorbide dinitrate

Isosorbide mononitrate

Isoxsuprine

L-Carnitine

Lidocaine

Lisinopril

Metaproterenol sulfate

Metaraminol bitartrate

Methoxamine hydrochloride

Metoprolol

Mexiletine

Cardiovascular Drugs (continued)

Mexiletine hydrochloride
Milrinone
Morphine SO$_4$
Nadolol
Nifedipine
Nitroglycerine 2% ointment
Nitroprusside
Phenoxybenzamine hydrochloride
Phentolamine
Phenylephrine
Phenytoin
Pimobendan
Prazosin
Procainamide
Propantheline bromide
Propranolol
Quinidine
Sotalol
Spironolactone/hydrochlorothiazide
Streptokinase
Taurine
Terbutaline
Tocainide
Verapamil hydrochloride
Warfarin

Dermatological Drugs (Topical, Cutaneous)

Acitretin
Aloe vera cream
Alpha-keri
Amitraz
Auranofin
Aurothioglucose
Benzoyl peroxide
Captan powder 50%
Chlorhexidine 0.5%
Chlorpheniramine
Clemastine
Clofazimine
Clomipramine
Clotrimazole
Dapsone
Derm Caps

Dermatological Drugs (Topical, Cutaneous) *(continued)*

Diethylstilbestrol
Diphenhydramine hydrochloride
Doramectin
Essential fatty acids
Etretinate
Fluoxymesterone
Gentamicin
Griseofulvin
Hydroxyzine
Isotretinoin
Lime sulfur suspension
Mafenide 10%
Melatonin
Methylprednisolone acetate
Miconazole
Montelukast
Nystatin
Omega fatty acids
Pentoxifylline
Phenobarbital
Polymyxin B

Potassium iodide
Povidone-iodine
Prednisolone
Silver nitrate solution 0.5%
Silver sulfadiazine
Sodium iodide 20%
Terbinafine
Terfenadine
Testosterone propionate
Tretinoin
Trimeprazine
Trimeprazine plus prednisone
Vitamin A
Vitamin E

Electrolyte Fluids/Volume Expanders

Calcium citrate
Dextran 40, 70
Dextrose 5%, 50%
Hemoglobin
Hetastarch
Hydroxyethyl starch

Electrolyte Fluids/Volume Expanders *(continued)*

Hypertonic saline
L-Deprenyl
Lactated Ringer's solution
Magnesium citrate
Magnesium sulfate
Phosphate sodium or potassium
Polyethylene glycol electrolyte solution
Potassium chloride
Sodium bicarbonate
Sodium chloride
Sodium chloride 7.5%
Sodium phosphate

Endocrine/Metabolic/Reproductive Drugs

Acarbose
Altrenogest
Aluminum carbonate gel
Bromocriptine mesylate
Cabergoline
Calcitonin
Calcitriol

Calcium gluconate 10%
Carbimazole
Chlorpropamide
Cholecalciferol
Chorionic gonadotropin
Clomiphene citrate
Cloprostenol
Colony-stimulating factor
Cortisone acetate
Danazol
Demeclocycline
Deoxycorticosterone acetate, pivalate
Deprenyl
Desmopressin acetate
Dexamethasone
Diazoxide
Diethylstilbestrol
1,25-dihydroxyvitamin D_3
Epostane
Erythropoietin
Estradiol cypioniate

Endocrine/Metabolic/Reproductive Drugs *(continued)*

Etidronate disodium
Finasteride
Fludrocortisone
Fluoxymesterone
Folinic acid
Follicle-stimulating hormone
Gemfibrozil
Glipizide
Glucagon
Glyburide
Gonadotropin-releasing hormone
Gonadorelin
Graunlocyte colony stimulating factor
Growth hormone (somatotropin)
Hydrochlorothiazide
Insulin, lente
Insulin, NPH
Insulin, PZI
Insulin, regular
Insulin, ultralente
Iodine

Ipodate
Ketoconazole
Levothyroxine T_4
Liothyronine T_3
Luteinizing hormone
Lysine-8-vasopressin
Medroxyprogesterone acetate
Megestrol acetate
Metapyrone
Metformin
Methimazole
Methyltestosterone
Mibolerone
Mifepristone
Mitotane
Oxytocin
Phosphate sodium or potassium
Prednisolone acetate
Propylthiouracil
Prostaglandin F_2 alpha
Sodium polystyrene sulfonate
Somatotropin
Spironolactone/hydrochlorothiazide

Endocrine/Metabolic/Reproductive Drugs *(continued)*

Tamoxifen
Testosterone cypionate
Testosterone ethanate
Testosterone methyl
Thyrotropin
L-Thyroxine, T_4
Triiodothyronine T_3, liothyronine
Urofollitropin
Vanadium
Vasopressin, aqueous
Vasopressin, tannate in oil
Vitamin D_3, calcitriol

Gastrointestinal Drugs

Aluminum magnesium hydroxide
Aminopentamide
6-Aminosalicylic acid
Apomorphine
Aprotinin
Ascorbic acid
Atropine

Bisacodyl
Bismuth subsalicylate, subcarbonate
Cascara sagrada
Castor oil
Chlordiazepoxide-clidinium
Chlorpromazine
Cholestyramine
Cimetidine
Cisapride
Colchicine
Cyclizine
Cyproheptadine hydrochloride
Dactinomycin
Darbazine
Dehydrocholic acid
Dexpanthenol
Diazepam
Dicyclomine
Dimenhydrinate
Dioctyl sulfosuccinate
Diphenoxylate hydrochloride
Docusate calcium, sodium

Gastrointestinal Drugs *(continued)*

Emetine
Famotidine
Flumazenil
Flunixin meglumine
Flurazepam
Glutamine
Glycerine enema
Glycopyrrolate
Isopropamide/prochlorperazine
Kaolin/pectin
Lactulose
Lactilol
Loperamide
Magnesium citrate
Magnesium hydroxide
Magnesium sulfate
Meclizine
Medium-chain triglycerides
Mesalamine
Metamucil
Methylcellulose
Methscopolamine

Metoclopramide
Metronidazole
Milk thistle (silymarin)
Mineral oil
Misoprostol
Nizatidine
Olsalazine
Omeprazole
Ondansetron
Opium tincture
Oxazepam
Pancreatic enzyme
Pancreatin
Paregoric
D-Penicillamine
Perphenizine
Phenobarbital
Prednisolone
Prochlorperazine
Promethazine hydrochloride
Propantheline bromide
Prucalopride
Psyllium

Gastrointestinal Drugs (continued)

Ranitidine hydrochloride
S-adenyosyl methionine
Scopolomine
Senna
Silymarin
Sorbital
Sucralfate
Sulfasalazine
Sulfobromophthalein sodium
Tetramine
Thiethylperazine
Triflupromazine
Trimethobenzamide
Ursodeoxycholic acid (ursodiol)
Viokase
Zinc acetate
Zinc sulfate

Immunomodulator/Cytotoxic/Anticancer Agents

Acemannan
Actinomycin D
Asparaginase
Auranofin
Aurothioglucose
Azathioprine
Bleomycin
Busulfan
Carboplatin
Carmustine
Chlorambucil
Cisplatin
Cyclophosphamide
Cyclosporine
Cytarabine
Cytosine arabinoside
Dacarbazine
Dactinomycin
Dexamethasone
Doxorubicin
5-Fluorouracil
Gamma globulin
Gold sodium thiomalate
Hydroxyurea

Immunomodulator/Cytotoxic/Anticancer Agents *(continued)*

Interferon α_2
Isofamide
L-Asparaginase
Lactoferrin
Lobaplatin
Lomustine
Lufeneron/milbemycin
Mebendazole
Mechlorethamine hydrochloride
Melphalan
6-Mercaptopurine
Methotrexate sodium
Methylprednisolone acetate
Mithramycin
Mitoxantrone
Mycobacterial cell wall extract
Neupogen
Nicotinamide (vitamin B_3)
Octreotide acetate
Paclitaxel
Pentoxifylline

Procarbazine hydrochloride
Propionibacterium acnes
Staphage lysate
Staphylococcal A
Streptozocin
Thioguanine
Thiotepa
Triamcinolone
Triethylene thiophosphoramide
Vinblastine
Vincristine

Neurological Drugs

Aminocaproic acid
Bromide, potassium or sodium
Carbamazepine
Clonazapam
Clorazepate (sustained release)
Clorazepate dipotassium
Dexamethasone
Dextroamphetamine
Diazepam

Neurological Drugs *(continued)*

Dimethyl sulfoxide 40%
Diphenylhydantoin
Divalproex sodium
Domperidone
Edrophonium chloride
Ethosuximide
Euthanasia solution
Felbamate
Flumazenil
Gaba pentin
Guaifenesin
Imipramine
Iohexol
Iopamidol
Levetiracetam
Mannitol 20%
Mephenytoin
Mepivacaine
Methocarbamol
Methylphenidate
Methyprednisolone sodium succinate

Nalbuphine
Neostigmine
Pentobarbital
Phenobarbital
Phenytoin
Prednisolone
Primidone
Protriptyline
Pyridostigmine bromide
Sufentanil
Tiletamine
Tolazoline
Valproic acid
Yohimbine

Ophthalmic Drugs

Acetazolamide
Antazoline 0.5%
Betamethasone
Cromolyn sodium 4%
Cyclosporine ophthalmic 1-2%
Dichlorphenamide

Ophthalmic Drugs *(continued)*

Disodium EDTA
Ethoxzolamide
Flunixin meglumine
Flurbiprofen
Gentamicin SO_4 0.1%
Glucose 40% ophthalmic
Glycerin
Idoxuridine
Mannitol 20%
Methazolamide
Methylprednisolone acetate
Miconazole
Natamycin
Physostigmine
Pilocarpine 1% ophthalmic solution
Prednisolone
Sodium chloride 5%
Suprofen 1% ophthalmic solution
Taurine
Triamcinolone ophthalmic solution
Trifluridine ophthalmic solution

Paralytic Agents

Atracurium besylate
Pancuronium bromide
Succinylcholine
Vecuronium bromide

Respiratory Drugs

Albuterol
Aminophylline
Budesonide
Butorphanol
Chlorpheniramine
Dextromethorphan
Doxapram
Ephedrine
Epinephrine
Fluticasone propionate
Furosemide
Hydrochlorothiazide
Hydrocodone bitartrate
Isoproterenol
Montelukast
Noscapine

Respiratory Drugs *(continued)*

Oxtriphylline
Prednisolone
Pseudoephedrine
Rutin
Spironolactone
Terbutaline
Theophylline
Theophylline sustained-release
Zafirlukast

Tranquilizers/Anesthetics/Analgesics/Antagonists

Acepromazine
Alfentanil
Atipamazole
Benzocaine
Bupivacaine hydrochloride
Buprenorphine
Butorphanol
Cetacaine
Chlorpromazine
Codeine
Diazepam

Domperidone
Enflurane
Ethylisobutrazine hydrochloride
Etomidate
Fentanyl citrate
Fentanyl/droperidol
Halothane
Isoflurane
Ketamine hydrochloride
Ketoroiac tromethamine
Levallorphan
Meclofenamic acid
Medetomidine hydrochloride
Meperidine hydrochloride
Methohexital
Methoxyflurane
Midazolam
Morphine SO_4
Nalbuphine
Nalmefene
Nalorphine hydrochloride
Naloxone hydrochloride

Tranquilizers/Anesthetics/Analgesics/Antagonists *(continued)*

Naltrexone
Oxymorphone
Pentazocine
Pentobarbital
Phenobarbital
Promethazine hydrochloride
Propiomazine
Propofol
Sodium thiopental
Sufentanil
Thiamylal sodium
Thiopental sodium
Tiletamine
Tolazoline
Xylazine
Yohimbine

Renoactive/Urinary Tract Drugs

Acetohydroxamic acid
Allopurinol
Aluminum hydroxide

Ammonium chloride
Ascorbic acid
Baclofen
Bethanechol
Calcitriol
Calcium citrate
Cyclothiazide
Dantrolene
Diazepam
Dicyclomine
Diethylstilbestrol
Dopamine hydrochloride
Ephedrine
Erythropoietin
Ethacrynic acid
Flavoxate
Furosemide
Imipramine
Isometheptene
Jenotone
Mannitol 20%
Magestrol acetate

Renoactive/Urinary Tract Drugs *(continued)*

2-Mercaptopropronyl glycine
Mesna
Methanimine hippurate
Methanamine mandelate
Dl-Methionine
Nandrolone decanoate
Oxybutinin
D-Penicillamine
Phenoxybenzamine hydrochloride
Phenylpropanolamine hydrochloride
Potassium citrate
Prednisolone
Propantheline bromide
Pseudoephedrine
Racemethionine
Sodium bicarbonate
Sodium chloride
Spironolactone
Stanozolol
Testosterone cypionate
Testosterone propionate
Tiopronin
Triamterene
Urea

Vitamins/Mineral/Supplements

Ascorbic acid
Brewer's yeast
Calcium (and calcium salts)
L-Carnitine
Cyanocobalamine
Dihydrotachysterol
1, 25-dihydroxyvitamin D_3
Ergocalciferol
Ferrous sulfate
Folic acid
Levocarnitine
Phytomenadione (Vitamin K_1)
Potassium chloride
Potassium gluconate
Retinol (Vitamin A)
Riboflavin (Vitamin B_2)
Sodium bicarbonate

Vitamins/Mineral/Supplements *(continued)*

Sodium chloride

Taurine

Thiamine (vitamin B_1)

Vitamin A

Vitamin B_1

Vitamin B_2 (riboflavin)

Vitamin B_{12}

Vitamin B complex

Vitamin C

Vitamin D, cholecalciferol, dihydrotachysterol

Vitamin D_2, ergocalciferol

Vitamin D_3, calcitriol, 1,25-dihydroxyvitamin D_3

Vitamin E

Vitamin K_1, phytomenadione

Zinc methionine

Zinc sulfate

Appendix B: Alphabetical Listing of Drugs by Generic and Proprietary Name and Source

Products listed in this appendix were selected based on their widespread availability and trade name recognition. Therefore, not all trade products have been included. An attempt has been made to include at least one commercial product that is available in the United States for each drug. Inclusion of a drug in this formulary does not guarantee its commercial availability. Likewise, dosing forms may be outdated by the time of the formulary's printing. The availability of commercial products is dynamic. Sources reviewed for evidence of availability included the Food and Drug Administration's (FDA) publically available Green or Orange Books, which delineate currently approved veterinary (animal) or human drugs, respectively. For veterinary drugs, the FDA also provides a list of drugs that have been voluntarily withdrawn. This list was also consulted during the preparation of this formulary to determine availability. Even if a drug was withdrawn, it may still be retained in the formulary because it may be obtained through compounding pharmacies. Clinicians are reminded that prescribing a compounded drug should be a patient-driven effort such that an individual patient's needs are met. Compounding when a commercially available drug is available that will meet the patient's needs is considered illegal in some states and is not an FDA-recognized practice. Further, prescribing compounded products that mimic commercial products is a major disincentive for animal divisions of pharmaceutical companies who make the decision to pursue approval of a drug in dogs or cats. Recovery of research, development, and market costs for products with a compounded version available is often only slowly realized because of the small population targeted by approved animal drugs. Note that only FDA-approved and United States Pharmacopeia (USP)-recognized dosing forms are listed in the formulary. Compounded preparations (e.g., transdermal gels, chews) are not specifically delineated partly because of the absence of scientific evidence supporting safe and effective use of such products. Compounded products undergo no federally mandated assessment of quality, safety, or efficacy. As such, compounded products used in leau of approved fixed dosing forms have greater risk of either therapeutic failure or toxicity. Therapeutic failure is probably of greater risk than toxicity. Veterinarians may wish to become familiar with the Pharmacy Compounding Accreditation Board (www.pcab.com) in their efforts to prescribe quality compounded products.

Sources for other unapproved products used as drugs (e.g., dietary supplements, either animal or human, including botanicals, herbs, and other "novel ingredients") are generally not provided. An exception is made for those products supported by scientific evidence of therapeutic efficacy. Dietary supplements undergo no federally mandated premarket assessment for quality, safety, or efficacy. Quality of some dietary supplements may be profoundly impaired. The Web site www.consumerlab.com may be a reasonable resource to find quality, commercially available novel ingredients. Species of approval is indicated for all listed drugs.

An attempt has been made to indicate whether or not a generic drug is available by indicating the brand versus proprietary name. The Orange Book, www.fda.gov/cder/ob/, and the Green Book, www.fda.gov/cvm/Green_Book/section22008.pdf, can be consulted to find generic sources for human or veterinary drugs, respectively. Generic products are approved by the FDA and must be proven to be equally bioavailable (similar rate and extent of absorption) and bioequivalent/pharmaceutically equivalent (i.e., same strength, dosing form, presence of active and inert ingredients) to the pioneer (or other generic) drug that the generic drug is mimicking. Most generic drugs included in this formulary are generic human products and the test for similar bioavailability in humans does not necessarily equate to similar bioavailability in the target species, unless specifically tested in that species.

Approved human products generally are chosen as the representative proprietary name if an animal approval exists, unless the human version is more available or convenient. Although an attempt was made to identify all products that have animal approval, some products may have been missed. Products approved in animals other than cats and dogs are included when the drug is not available in a preparation approved for small animals or humans.

Over-the-counter (OTC) products often were not included in the formulary because of the lack of information. Clinicians should be aware that the generic products associated with an OTC product can change. For example, Kaopectate now consists of several different products, a number of which contain bismuth subsalicylate. Clients should be directed to OTC products based on the generic content.

Occasionally, drugs available in countries other than the United States are included in the formulary (e.g., trilostane at the time of publication). Although pharmacists may be able to compound such drugs, their importation into the United States requires permission from the FDA's Office of Compliance. Note that among the reasons the FDA does not approve importation of foreign products is their inability to assure the quality of the drugs themselves or active (or inactive) ingredients imported in bulk. Compounding pharmacies should be queried to assure the quality of substances used for compounded preparations.

Generic Name	Proprietary Name	Strength	Form	Source	Approval
Acarbose	Precose	25 mg, 50 mg, 100 mg	Tablet	Bayer	3
Acemannan	Carrisyn	NI	Injectable	Carrington Laboratories	B
Acepromazine maleate	Acepromazine, others	10 mg/mL	Injectable	Boehringer Ingelheim, others	1
Acepromazine maleate	Acepromazine, others	10 mg, 25 mg	Tablet	Boehringer Ingelheim, others	1
Acepromazine maleate	PromAce	5 mg, 10 mg, 25 mg	Tablet	Fort Dodge	1, 2
Acepromazine maleate	PromAce	10 mg/mL	Injectable	Fort Dodge	1
Acetaminophen	Tylenol, generic	65mg-650 mg	Rectal suppository, tablet	McNeil Consumer	OTC
Acetazolamide	Diamox	500 mg extended release	Capsule	Lederle	3
Acetazolamide	Diamox	125 mg, 250 mg	Tablet	Mutual Pharmaceuticals	3
Acetazolamide	Diamox	500 mg/vial	Injectable	Barr	3
Acetohydroxamic acid	Lithostat	250 mg	Tablet	Mission Pharma	3
Acetylcysteine	Acetylcysteine	10%, 20% solution	Inhalation, oral solution	Bedford	3
Acetylcysteine	Acetylcysteine	10%, 20% solution	Inhalation, oral solution	Hospira	3
Acetylcysteine	Mucomyst	10%, 20% solution	Inhalation, oral solution	Apothecon	3

Generic Name	Proprietary Name	Strength	Form	Source	Approval
Acetylcysteine	Acetadote	200 mg/mL (6 g/30 mL)	Injectable-IV	Cumberland Pharmaceuticals	3
Acetylsalicylic acid	Aspirin, generic	Multiple strengths	Tablet	Bayer, others	OTC
Actinomycin D (dactinomycin)	Cosmegen	0.5 mg vial	Injectable	Merck	3
Activated charcoal	Actidose-Aqua	12.5 g/60 mL	Oral slurry		OTC
Activated charcoal	Charco-caps	260 mg	Capsule		OTC
Acyclovir	Zovirax	200 mg, 400 mg, 800 mg	Capsule	GlaxoSmithKline	3
Acyclovir	Zovirax	5%	Ointment, cream	GlaxoSmithKline	3
Acyclovir	Zovirax	40 mg/mL	Oral solution	GlaxoSmithKline	3
Acyclovir	Zovirax	500 mg, 1 g	Injectable	GlaxoSmithKline	3
Acyclovir (valacyclovir hydrochloride)	Valtrex	500 mg, 1g	Tablet	GlaxoSmithKline	3
Albendazole	Valbazen	30% paste, 4.55%, 11.4% solution	Oral solution	Pfizer	4
Albendazole	Albenza	200 mg	Tablet	GlaxoSmithKline	3
Albuterol	Proventil	2 mg, 4 mg extended release	Tablet	Schering-Plough	3
Albuterol	Ventolin	2 mg/5 mL	Syrup	GlaxoSmithKline	

Generic Name	Proprietary Name	Strength	Form	Source	Approval
Albuterol	Proventil	90 μg/17g, 6.7 g canisters	Inhalant	3M	3
Albuterol	Proventil	0.083 or 0.5%	Inhalant solution	3M	3
Albuterol	Proventil	2 mg, 4 mg, or 8 mg extended release	Tablet	Pliva	3
Albuterol	Proventil	2 mg/5 mL	Syrup	Hi Tech Pharmaceuticals	3
Albuterol	Albuterol sulfate	2 mg, 4 mg	Tablet	Mutual Pharmaceuticals	3
Albuterol	Albuterol sulfate	0.083%, 0.5%	Inhalant solution	Bausch and Lomb	3
Albuterol (levalbuterol hydrochloride)	Xopenoex	0.0103, 0.021, 0.042, or 0.25%	Inhalant solution	Sepracor	3
Alfentanil	Alfenta	500 μg/mL	Injectable	Novation	3
Allopurinol	Allopurinol	100 mg, 300 mg	Tablet	Mutual Pharmaceuticals	3
Allopurinol	Allopurinol	500 mg base/vial	Injectable	Bedford Laboratories	3
Aloe vera cream	Aloe	NA	Topical	NI	C
Aloe vera cream	Dermaide, Aloe	NA	Topical	NI	C
Alprazolam	Xanax	0.25 mg, 0.5 mg, 1 mg, 2 mg	Tablet	Pharmacia and Upjohn	3
Alprazolam	Xanax XR	0.5 mg, 1 mg, 2 mg, 3 mg extended release	Tablet	Pharmacia and Upjohn	3

Generic Name	Proprietary Name	Strength	Form	Source	Approval
Alprazolam	Niravam	0.25 mg, 0.5 mg, 1 mg, 2 mg orally disintegrating	Tablet	Schwarz Pharma	3
Alprazolam	Alprazolam	1 mg/mL	Oral concentrate	Roxane	3
Altrenogest	Regu-Mare, Matrix	2.2 mg/mL (0.22%) in 150 or 1000 mL vials	In oil	Intervet	4
Aluminum carbonate gel	Basalgel	500 mg	Capsule	Wyeth	4
Aluminum hydroxide	Amphojel, others	320 mg/5 mL	Oral suspension	Wyeth-Ayerst, others	3, OTC
Aluminum hydroxide	Amphojel	300 mg, 600mg	Tablet	Wyeth-Ayerst	3
Aluminum hydroxide	Foam Coat	20 mg, 80 mg	Tablet	Guardian Drug	OTC
Amantadine	Symmatrel	100 mg	Tablet	Multiple	3
Amikacin	Amikin	50 mg/mL, 250 mg/mL	Injectable	Apothecon	1
Aminocaproic acid (EACA)	Amicar	1.25 mg/5 ml., 500 mg	Syrup, tablet	Xanodyne Pharmaceuticals	3
Aminocaproic acid	Amicar	250 mg/mL	Injectable	Xanodyne Pharmaceuticals	3
Aminopentamide	Centrine	0.2 mg	Tablet	Fort Dodge	1, 2
Aminopentamide	Centrine	0.5 mg/mL	Injectable	Fort Dodge	1, 2
Aminophylline	Aminophylline	1.5 grains, 3 grains	Tablet	Global Pharmaceutical	3

Generic Name	Proprietary Name	Strength	Form	Source	Approval
Aminophylline	Aminophylline, others	100 mg, 200 mg	Tablet	West-Ward, others	3
Aminophylline	Aminophylline	105 mg/5 mL	Oral solution	Roxane	3
Aminophylline	Aminophylline	100 mg/100 mL, 200 mg/100 mL, 25 mg/mL	Injectable	Hospira	3
Aminophylline	Truphylline	250 mg, 500 mg	Rectal suppository	G and W Labs	3
Amiodarone	Cordarone	50 mg/mL	Injectable	Wyeth Pharmaceuticals	3
Amiodarone	Amiodarone hydrochloride	100, 200, 300, 400 mg	Tablet	Taro	3
Amiodarone	Pacerone	100, 200 mg	Tablet	Upsher-Smith	3
Amitraz	Mitaban	19.90%	Topical	Pharmacia and Upjohn	1
Amitriptyline hydrochloride	Amitriptyline hydrochloride, generic	10 mg, 25 mg, 50 mg, 75 mg, 100 mg, 150 mg	Tablet	Mutual Pharmaceuticals, others	3
Amitriptyline hydrochloride	Anapryl	2 mg, 5 mg, 10 mg, 15 mg, 30 mg	Tablet	Pfizer	1
Amlodipine	Norvasc	2.5 mg, 5 mg, 10 mg (base)	Tablet	Pfizer	3
Ammonium chloride	Ammonium chloride in plastic container	5 mEq/mL	Injectable	Hospira	3
Amoxicillin trihydrate	Amoxi tabs, generic	50 mg, 100 mg, 150 mg, 200 mg, 400 mg	Tablet	Pfizer, others	1, 2
Amoxicillin trihydrate	Amoxi-drops	50 mg/mL	Oral solution	Pfizer	1, 2

Generic Name	Proprietary Name	Strength	Form	Source	Approval
Amoxicillin trihydrate	Amoxi-Inject	3 g	Injectable	Pfizer	1, 2
Amoxicillin/clavulanic acid	Clavamox	50 mg, 100 mg, 200 mg, 300 mg/12.5 mg, 25 mg, 50 mg, 75 mg	Tablet	Pfizer	1, 2
Amphetamine SO_4	Adderall	1.25 mg, 1.875 mg, 2.5 mg, 3.125 mg, 3.75 mg, 5 mg, 7.5 mg	Tablet	Shire Richwood	3
Amphetamine SO_4	Adderall XR	2.5 mg, 5 mg, 7.5 mg	Tablet	Shire Richwood	3
Amphotericin B	Fungizone	50 mg/vial	Injectable	Apothecon	3
Amphotericin B	Fungizone	3%	Topical cream	Apothecon	3
Amphotericin B	Fungizone	3%	Topical lotion	Apothecon	3
Amphotericin B lipid complex	Abelcet	5 mg/mL	Injectable	Liposome	3
Amphotericin B lipid complex	Amphotec	50, 100 mg/vial	Injectable, lipid complex	Three Rivers Pharms	3
Amphotericin B liposome	AmBisome	50 mg/vial	Injectable, liposomal	Astellas	3
Ampicillin	Omnipen, generic	125 mg, 250 mg	Tablet	Fort Dodge, others	1, 3
Ampicillin	Principen	25 mg/mL, 50 mg/mL, 100 mg/mL	Oral solution	Apothecon	3

Generic Name	Proprietary Name	Strength	Form	Source	Approval
Ampicillin	Princillin	250 mg, 500 mg	Capsule	Apothecon	3
Ampicillin/sublactam	Unasyn	125 mg, 250 mg, 500 mg, 1 g, 2 g, 10 g/vial	Injectable	Sandoz	3
Ampicillin trihydrate	Polyflex	50 mg/mL, 100 mg/mL, 200 mg/mL	Injectable	Fort Dodge	1, 2
Amprolium	Corid	20%	Powder	Merial	4
Amrinone	Inocor	5 mg/mL	Injectable	Bedford	3
Antimony	Pentostam	NI	NI	NI	NI
Antivenin to Coral Snake	Coral (*Micrurus fulvius*)	NA	Injectable	Wyeth Laboratories	3, B
Antivenin to USA pit vipers	Crotilidae (polyvalent)	NA	Injectable	Wyeth Laboratories	3, B
Apomorphine	Apomorphine, generic	20 mg/2 mL, 30 mg/30 mL (10 mg/mL)	SC Injectable	Multiple	3
Aprotinin	Trasylol	10,000 IU/mL	Injectable	Bayer	3
Ascorbic acid	Ascorbicap	100 mg, 500 mg, others	Tablet, capsule	Multiple	D
Ascorbic acid	Cebione	100 mg, 500 mg, others	Tablet, capsule	Multiple	D
Ascorbic acid	Cecon	100 mg, 500 mg, others	Tablet, capsule	Multiple	D
Ascorbic acid	Vitamin C	100 mg, 500 mg, others	Tablet, capsule	Multiple	D

Generic Name	Proprietary Name	Strength	Form	Source	Approval
Asparaginase	Elspar	10,000 Units	Powder for injection	Merck	3
Astemizole	Hismanal	1 mg/mL or 10 mg	Syrup or tablet	McNeil Consumer Healthcare	5
Atenolol	Tenormin	25 mg, 50 mg, 100 mg	Tablet	AstraZeneca Pharms	3
Atenolol	Tenormin	0.5 mg/mL	Injectable	AstraZeneca Pharms	3
Atipamazole	Antisedan	5 mg/mL	Injectable	Orion	1
Atovaquaone	Mepron	150 mg/mL (750 mg/5 mL)	Oral solution	Glaxosmithkline	3
Atovaquaone	Mepron	250 mg/mL	Tablet	Glaxosmithkline	3
Atracurium besylate	Tracrium	10 mg/mL	Injectable	Hospira	3
Atropine	Atropen, generic	EQ 0.25 mg sulfate/0.3 mL, EQ 0.5, 1, 2 mg sulfate/0.7 mL	Injectable	Meridian Medical Technologies, others	3
Auranofin	Ridaura	3 mg	Capsule	Prometheus Labs	3
Aurothioglucose	Solganal	NI	Injectable	NI	3
Azathioprine	Imuran	50 mg	Tablet	Prometheus Labs	3
Azrithromycin	Zythromax	250 mg, 500 mg, 600 mg	Tablet	Pfizer	3
Azrithromycin	Zythromax	100 mg, 200 mg, 1 g	Oral solution (suspension)	Pfizer	3

Generic Name	Proprietary Name	Strength	Form	Source	Approval
Aztreonam	Azactam	500 mg/mL	Injectable	Pfizer	3
Aztreonam	Azactam	500 mg, 1 g/vial, 2 g/vial	Injectable	Bristol-Myers Squibb	3
Aztreonam	Azactam	20 mg/mL, 40 mg/mL	Injectable	Bristol-Myers Squibb	3
Baclofen	Lioresal	2000 μg/mL	Injectable	Novartis	3
Baclofen	Lioresal	10 mg, 20 mg	Tablet	Novartis	3
Baquiloprim/sulphameth-oxine or sulphadiamine	Dazikan, Zaquilan	NI	NI	NI	5
Beclomethasone diproprionate	Beconase AQ	0.042 mg diproprionate/spray	Metered nasal spray	GlaxoSmithKline	3
Beclomethasone diproprionate	Qvar 40/80	0.04 mg/puff, 0.08 mg/puff	Metered inhalation solution	3M	3
Benazepril	Fortekor	5 mg, 10 mg, 20 mg, 40 mg	Tablet	Novartis	1, 2, 3
Bendroflumethiazide	Corzide	5 mg, 40 mg, 80 mg	Tablet	King Pharmaceuticals	3
Betamethasone	Celestone	0.12 mg/mL	Oral solution	Schering-Plough	3
Betamethasone	Diprolene AF	0.05% base	Topical cream	Schering-Plough	3
Betamethasone	Diprolene	0.05% base	Topical gel	Schering-Plough	3
Betamethasone	Celestone	0.6 mg	Tablet	Schering-Plough	3

Generic Name	Proprietary Name	Strength	Form	Source	Approval
Betamethasone	Celestone phosphate	4 mg/mL	Injectable	Schering-Plough	3
Betamethasone acetate and sodium phosphate	Celestone soluspan	3 mg/mL; EQ 3 mg base/mL	Injectable	Schering-Plough	3
Bethanechol	Urecholine	5 mg, 10 mg, 25 mg, 50 mg	Tablet	Odyessey Pharms	3
Bisacodyl	Dulcolax	5 mg	Enteric coated tablet	Boehringer Ingelheim	3
Bismuth subsalicylate	Pepto-Bismol	Aspirin equivalent: 9 mg/mL, 18 mg/mL, 130 mg/tablet	Oral solution, tablet	Multiple	OTC
Bleomycin	Blenoxane	15 Units/vial, 30 Units/vial	Injectable	Bristol-Myers Squibb	3
Brewer's yeast	Brewer's yeast	NA			D
Bromide, potassium or sodium	NA	Not approved for use in the USA		ICN	5
Bromocriptine mesylate	Parlodel	EQ 2.5 mg base	Tablet	Novartis	3
Bromocriptine mesylate	Parlodel	EQ 5 mg base	Capsule	Novartis	3
Budesonide	Entocort EC, Entocard	3 mg (micronized)	Capsule	AstraZeneca	
Bunamidine	Scolaban	400 mg	Tablet	Schering-Plough	1, 2
Bupivacaine hydrochloride	Marcaine	0.25%. 0.5%, 0.75% with or without epinephrine	Injectable	Hospira	3
Bupivacaine hydrochloride	Marcaine	0.75%	Injectable, spinal	Hospira	3

Generic Name	Proprietary Name	Strength	Form	Source	Approval
Buprenorphine	Buprenex	0.3 mg/mL	Injectable	Reckitt Benckiser	3
Buprenorphine	Buprenex	EQ 2 mg, 8 mg base	Tablet, sublingual	Reckitt Benckiser	3
Buspirone	Buspar	5 mg, 10 mg, 15 mg, 30 mg	Tablet	Bristol-Myers Squibb	3
Busulfan	Myleran	2 mg	Tablet	GlaxoSmithKline	3
Busulfan	Busulfex	6 mg/mL	Injectable	ESP Pharma	3
Butamisole	Styquin	11 mg	Injectable	Cyanamid	1
Butorphanol	Torbutrol	0.5 mg/mL	Injectable	Fort Dodge	1
Butorphanol	Torbutrol	1 mg, 5 mg, 10 mg	Tablet	Fort Dodge	1
Butorphanol	Torbugesic	2 mg/mL	Injectable	Fort Dodge	2
Cabergoline	Dostinex	500 μg	Tablet	Pfizer	3
Calcitriol (Vitamin D^3)	Calcijex	0.001 mg/mL, 0.002 mg/mL	Injectable	Abbott	3
Calcitriol	Rocaltrol	0.25 μg, 0.5 μg	Capsule	Roche	3
Calcitriol	Rocaltrol	1 μg/mL	Oral solution	Roche	3
Calcium acetate	Phosphlo	169 mg	Tablet	Nabi	3

Generic Name	Proprietary Name	Strength	Form	Source	Approval
Calcium acetate	Phosphlo Gelcaps	169 mg	Capsule	Nabi	3
Calcium carbonate	Tums	200 mg, 300 mg, 400 mg, 500 mg elemental calcium	Tablet	SmithKline Beecham	OTC
Calcium chloride	Calcium chloride, generic	100 mg/mL	Injectable	Hospira, others	3
Calcium chloride	Calcium chloride	1 g/vial	Injectable	Bristol-Myers-Squibb	3
Calcium citrate	Calcium citrate	NE			
Calcium EDTA	Versenate	200 mg/mL	Injectable	3M	3
Calcium gluconate 10%	Calglucon	100 mg/mL	Injectable	Vortech Pharmaceuticals	3
Calcium lactate	Calphosan, generic	325 mg, 650 mg	Tablet	Eli Lilly, others	3
Calcium lactate	Calphosan	10 grains, 83.3 mg, 1000 mg	Tablet	Perrigo	3
Calcium lactate	Calphosan, generic	100 mg	Tablet	Schiff Products, others	3
Captan powder, 50%	Orthocide	50%	Powder		1
Captopril	Capoten	12.5 mg, 25 mg, 50 mg, 100 mg	Tablet	PAR Pharm	3
Carbamazepine	Epitol	100 mg, 200 mg, 400 mg	Tablet, chewable	Novartis	3
Carbamazepine	Epitol	200 mg	Tablet	Teva	3

Generic Name	Proprietary Name	Strength	Form	Source	Approval
Carbamazepine	Carbamazepine	100 mg, 200 mg	Tablet, chewable	Taro Pharmaceutical Industries	3
Carbamazepine	Tegretol	100 mg/5 mL	Oral suspension	Novartis	3
Carbenicillin	Geocillin	382 mg	Tablet	Pfizer	3
Carbenicillin indanyl sodium	Geopen	382 mg	Tablet	Pfizer	3
Carbimazole	Neo-Mercazole	Not approved for use in the USA			
Carboplatin	Paraplatin	50 mg/vial, 150 mg/vial, 450 mg/vial	Injectable	Bristol-Myers Squibb	3
Carmustine	BICNU	100 mg/vial	Injectable	Bristol-Myers Squibb	3
Carprofen	Rimadyl	25 mg, 75 mg, 100 mg	Tablet	Pfizer	3
Carprofen	Rimadyl	25 mg, 75 mg, 100 mg	Tablet, chewable	Pfizer	3
Carvedilol	Coreg, generic	3.125 mg, 6.25 mg, 12.5 mg, 25 mg	Tablet	GlaxoSmithKline	3
Cascara sagrada	Nature's Remedy, generic	100 mg, 325 mg	Tablet	Multiple	1, 2
Castor oil	Emulsoil, Neoloid, Purge	36.4%, 95%	Emulsion, oral liquid	OTC	OTC
Cefaclor	Ceclor	375 mg, 500 mg	Tablet, extended release	Teva	3
Cefaclor	Ceclor	125 mg/5 mL, 187 mg/5 mL, 250 mg/5 mL, 375 mg/5 mL	Powder for oral suspension	Ranbaxy	3

Generic Name	Proprietary Name	Strength	Form	Source	Approval
Cefaclor	Ceclor CD	125 mg, 187 mg, 250 mg, 375 mg	Tablet, chewable	Ranbaxy	3
Cefaclor	Raniclor	250 mg, 500 mg	Capsule	Ranbaxy	3
Cefadroxil	Cefaclor	1 g	Tablet	Ranbaxy	3
Cefadroxil	Cefadroxil	125 mg/5 mL, 250 mg/5 mL, 500 mg/5mL	Oral suspension	Ranbaxy	3
Cefadroxil	Cefadroxil	500 mg	Capsule	Ranbaxy	3
Cefamandole	Mandol	10 g/vial	Injectable	Lilly	3
Cefamandole	Mandol	1 g/vial, 2 g/vial	Injectable	Lilly	3
Cefazolin sodium	Ancef	10 mg/mL , 20 mg/mL	Injectable	Baxter Healthcare	3
Cefazolin sodium	Kefzol, generic	50 mg/50 mL, 100 mg/50 mL	Injectable	Multiple	1, 2
Cefovecin	Convenia	80 mg/mL	Injectable	Pfizer	1, 2
Cefepime	Maxipime	0.5 g/vial, 1 g/vial, 2 g/vial	Injectable	Bristol Meyers Squibb	3
Cefixime	Suprax	400 mg	Tablet	Lupin	3
Cefixime	Suprax	20 mg/mL	Oral solution	Lupin	3
Cefmetazole	Zefazone	20 mg/mL, 40 mg/mL, 1g, 2 g	Injectable	Pharmacia and Upjohn	3

Generic Name	Proprietary Name	Strength	Form	Source	Approval
Cefovecin	Convenia	80 mg/mL	Injectable	Pfizer	1, 2
Cefoperazone	Cefobid	EQ 1 g base/vial, 2 g base/vial, 10 g base/vial	Injectable	Pfizer	3
Cefoperazone	Cefobid in plastic container	EQ 20 mg base/vial, 40 mg base/vial	Injectable	Pfizer	3
Cefotaxime	Claforan	EQ 0.5 g/vial, 1 g/vial, 2 g/vial, 10 g/vial, 20 mg/mL, 40 mg/mL	Injectable	Aventis Pharmaceuticals	3
Cefotetan	Cefotan	EQ 1 g base/vial, 2 g base/vial, 10 g base/vial	Injectable	Astrazeneca Pharms	3
Cefotetan	Cefotan in plastic container	EQ 20 mg base/vial, 40 mg base/vial	Injectable	Astrazeneca Pharms	3
Cefoxitin sodium	Mefoxin in dextrose 5% in plastic container	EQ 20 mg/base/mL, 40 mg base/mL	Injectable	Merck	3
Cefoxitin sodium	Mefoxin in plastic container	1 g base/vial, 2 g base/vial, 10 g base/vial	Injectable	Merck	3
Cefpodoxime	Vantin	100 mg, 200 mg	Tablet	Pharmacia and Upjohn	3
Cefpodoxime	Vantin	10 mg/mL, 20 mg/mL	Oral solution	Pharmacia and Upjohn	3
Ceftazidime	Ceptaz	1 g/vial, 2 g/vial, 10 g/vial	Injectable	GlaxoSmithKline	3
Ceftiofur	Naxcel	50 mg/mL	Injectable	Pfizer	1
Ceftizoxime	Cefizox	EQ 1 g base/vial, 2 g base/vial, 10 g base/vial	Injectable	Astellas	3

Generic Name	Proprietary Name	Strength	Form	Source	Approval
Ceftizoxime	Cefizox in plastic container	EQ 20 mg base/vial, 40 mg base/vial	Injectable	Astellas	3
Ceftriaxone	Rocephin	20 mg/mL, 40 mg/mL, 0.25 g, 0.5 g, 1 g, 2 g, 10 g 7.5 g base/vial	Injectable	HLR	3
Cefuroxime	Cefuroxime	EQ 1.5 g base/vial, 7.5 g base/vial	Injectable	Teva	3
Cefuroxime	Cefuroxime axetil	125 mg, 250 mg, 500 mg	Tablet	Ranbaxy	3
Cefuroxime	Cefuroxime	EQ 750 mg base/vial	Injectable	TEVA	3
Cefuroxime	Cefuroxime sodium	EQ 750 mg base/vial	Injectable	Hanford GC	3
Cefuroxime	Cefuroxime sodium	EQ 1.5, 7.5 g base/vial	Injectable	AM Pharm Partners	3
Cefuroxime	Ceftin	125 mg/5 mL, 250 mg/5 mL	Injectable	GlaxoSmithKline	3
Cephadroxil	Duricef, others	500 mg	Capsule	Bristol-Meyers Squibb, others	3
Cephadroxil	Duricef, others	125 mg/mL, 250 mg/mL, 500 mg/mL	Oral solution	Bristol-Meyers Squibb, others	3
Cephalexin	Keflex, generic	250 mg, 500 mg	Capsule	Lilly, CEPH International, others	3
Cephalexin	Keflex, generic	25 mg/mL, 50 mg/mL, 100 mg/mL	Oral suspension	CEPH International, others	3
Cephalothin sodium	Keflin in plastic container	EQ 1 g base/vial, 2 g base/vial, 4 g base/vial	Injectable	Lilly	3

Generic Name	Proprietary Name	Strength	Form	Source	Approval
Cephalothin sodium	Cephalothin sodium	EQ 1 g base/vial, 2 g base/vial, 4 base/vial	Injectable	Bristol-Myers Squibb	3
Cephamandole		0.5 g/vial, 1 g/vial, 2 g/vial	Injectable	Mayne Pharma	3
Cephapirin	Cefadyl	500 mg, 1 g/vial, 2 g/vial, 4 g/vial	Injectable	Apothecon	3
Cephradine	Anspor	250 mg, 500 mg	Capsule	GlaxoSmithKline	3
Cephradine	Anspor	25 mg/mL, 50 mg/mL	Oral solution	GlaxoSmithKline	3
Cetacaine	Cetacaine	10 mg	Lozenge	NI	3
Cetacaine	Cetacaine	6.4%, 7.5%, 20%	Oral gel	NI	3
Cetacaine	Cetacaine	20%	Otic solution	NI	3
Cetacaine	Cetacaine	14%, 20%	Topical aerosol	NI	3
Cetacaine	Cetacaine	20%	Topical gel	NI	3
Cetrazine	Zyrtec	5 mg/5 mL	Oral syrup	Pfizer	3, OTC
Cetirizine hydrochloride	Zyrtec	5 mg, 10 mg	Tablet, chewable	Pfizer	4, OTC
Cetirizine hydrochloride	Zyrtec	5 mg, 10 mg	Tablet, chewable	Pfizer	5, OTC

Generic Name	Proprietary Name	Strength	Form	Source	Approval
Cetirizine hydrochloride (pseudoepedrine hydrochloride)	Zyrtec-D 12 Hour	5 mg (120 mg)	Tablet, extended release	Pfizer	6, OTC
Charcoal, activated	Toxiban, generic	15 g/72 mL-50 g/240 mL	Oral suspension, granule	Multiple	OTC
Chlorambucil	Leukeran	2 mg	Tablet	GlaxoSmithKline	3
Chloramphenicol	Chloromycetin	250 mg	Capsule	Compound	3
Chloramphenicol	Chloromycetin hydrocortisone	100 mg, 250 mg, 500 mg	Tablet	Compound	3
Chloramphenicol sodium succinate	Chloramphenicol sodium succinate, generic	EQ 1 g base/vial	Injectable	GlaxoSmithKline	3
Chlordiazepoxide	Librium	5, 10, 25 mg	Tablet	Multiple sources including generic	
Chlordiazepoxide/clidinium	Librax	5 mg/2.5 mg	Capsule	Roche	3
Chlorhexidine acetate	Novaldent	0.10%	Dental solution	TEVA	1, 2, 3
Chlorhexidine acetate	Periochip	2.5 mg	Dental tablet	Dexcel Pharma	3
Chlorhexidine gluconate	C.E.T.	0.12%	Dental solution	TEVA	1, 2, 3
Chlorhexidine diacetate	Nolvasan	2%	Solution	Fort Dodge	
Chlorothiazide	Diuril	250 mg, 500 mg	Tablet	Merck	3

Generic Name	Proprietary Name	Strength	Form	Source	Approval
Chlorothiazide	Diuril	50 mg/mL	Oral solution	Merck	3
Chlorothiazide	Diuril	500 mg/vial	Injectable	Merck	3
Chlorpheniramine	Chlor-Trimetron Allergy 8 and 12 Hour	8 mg, 12 mg extended release	Tablet	Schering-Plough	OTC
Chlorpheniramine	Chlorpheniramine	10 mg/mL	Injectable	Steris	3
Chlorpheniramine	Chlorpheniramine Maleate, generic	2 mg, 4 mg	Tablet	Multiple	OTC
Chlorpheniramine	Aller-Chlor	2 mg/5 mL (118 mL bottles)	Oral suspension	Rugby	OTC
Chlorpromazine	Thorazine	25 mg, 100 mg	Rectal suppository	SmithKline Beecham	3
Chlorpromazine	Thorazine Spansules	30 mg, 75 mg, 150 mg extended release	Capsule	SmithKline Beecham	3
Chlorpromazine	Thorazine	10 mg, 25 mg, 50 mg, 100 mg, 200 mg	Capsule	SmithKline Beecham	3
Chlorpromazine	Thorazine	25 mg/mL	Injectable	SmithKline Beecham	3
Chlorpromazine	Thorazine	2 mg/mL (120 mL bottles) 30 mg/mL (120 mL bottles) 100 mg/mL (60 and 240 mL bottles)	Oral solution	SmithKline Beecham	3
Chlorpropamide	Diabenese	100 mg, 250 mg	Tablet	Pfizer	3

Generic Name	Proprietary Name	Strength	Form	Source	Approval
Cholecalciferol	Fosamax Plus D	2,800 IU (EQ 70 mg base)	Tablet	Merck	3
Cholestyramine	Questran Light	EQ 4 g resin/packet	Powder for oral suspension	Bristol-Myers Squibb	3
Cholestyramine	Questran Light	EQ 4 g resin/scoopful	Powder for oral suspension	Bristol-Myers Squibb	3
Chondroitin sulfate/ glucosamine/ascorbate/ manganese	Cosequin, generic	250 mg/200 mg/ 33 mg/5 mg or 500 mg/ 400 mg/66 mg/10 mg	Capsule	Nutramax Laboratories, others	D
Chorionic gonadotropin	Follutein	10,000 USP/vial	Injectable	Butler	4
Cimetidine	Tagamet, generic	200 mg, 300 mg, 400 mg, 800 mg	Tablet	SmithKline Beecham, others	3
Cimetidine	Tagamet	150 mg/mL, 300 mg/50mL 0.9%NaCl	Injectable	SmithKline Beecham	3
Cimetidine	Tagamet	300 mg/5 mL	Oral solution	SmithKline Beecham	3
Ciprofloxacin	Cipro	200 mg in 20 mL vials, 400 mg in 40 mL vials	Injectable	Bayer	3
Ciprofloxacin	Cipro	5 g/100 mL, 10 g/100 mL	Oral solution	Bayer	3
Ciprofloxacin	Cipro	100 mg, 250 mg, 500 mg, 750 mg	Tablet	Bayer	3
Ciprofloxacin	Cipro HC	0.2% base, 1%	Otic solution	Alcon	3
Ciprofloxacin	Cipro	0.30%	Ophthalmic ointment/drops	Alcon	3

Generic Name	Proprietary Name	Strength	Form	Source	Approval
Cisapride	Propulsid	Removed from U.S. Market. May be available from compounding pharmacy	Removed from U.S. Market	Janssen (Discontinued)	3
Cisplatin	Platinol-AQ	1mg/mL in 50 mL, 100 mL, 200 mL multidose vials	Injectable	Bristol-Myers Oncology	3
Clarithromycin	Biaxin	25 mg/mL, 50 mg/mL in 50 mL and 100 mL	Oral solution	Abbott	3
Clarithromycin	Biaxin	500 mg extended release	Tablet	Abbott	3
Clarithromycin	Biaxin	250 mg, 500 mg	Tablet	Abbott	3
Clemastine	Tavist	1.34 mg, 2.68 mg	Tablet	Novartis	3
Clemastine	Tavist	0.67 mg/5 mL in 118 mL	Oral solution	Novartis	3
Clenbuterol	Vetipulmin	72.5 μg/mL in 100 mL, 330 mL, 460 mL bottles	Oral syrup	Boehringer Ingelheim	4
Clindamycin	Antirobe	25 mg, 75 mg, 150 mg, 300 mg	Capsule	Pfizer	1, 2
Clindamycin	Antirobe Aquadrops	25 mg/mL in 30 mL bottles	Oral solution	Pfizer	1, 2
Clindamycin	Cleocin Phosphate	150 mg/mL	Injectable	Pharmacia and Upjohn	3
Clindamycin	Cleocin Pediatric	75 mg/5 mL in 100 mL bottles	Oral solution	Pharmacia and Upjohn	3
Clindamycin	Cleocin	100 mg clindamycin/ 2.5 g suppository	Rectal suppository	Pharmacia and Upjohn***	3

Generic Name	Proprietary Name	Strength	Form	Source	Approval
Clindamycin	Cleocin	2%	Vaginal cream	Pharmacia and Upjohn	3
Clofazimine	Lamprene	50 mg	Capsule	Novartis	3
Clomiphene citrate	Clomid	50 mg	Tablet	Aventis Pharmaceuticals	3
Clomipramine	Anafranil	25 mg, 50 mg, 75 mg	Capsule	Novartis	3
Clomipramine	Clomicalm	20 mg, 40 mg, 80 mg	Tablet	Novartis	1
Clonazepam	Klonopin, generic	0.5 mg, 1 mg, 2 mg	Tablet	Roche, others	3
Clonidine	Duraclon	100 µg/mL or 500 µg/mL	Epidural injection	Elan	3
Clonidine	Catapres	0.1 mg, 0.2 mg, 0.3 mg	Tablet	BI, generic	3
Cloprostenol	Estrumate	250 µg/mL in 20 mL vials		Schering-Plough	3
Clorazepate	Tranxene	3.75 mg, 7.5 mg, 11.25 mg, 15 mg	Tablet	Abbott	3
Clorazepate	Tranxene	11.25 mg, 22.5 mg sustained release	Tablet	Abbott	3
Clotrimazole	Veltrim	1%	Cream	Bayer	1, 2
Clotrimazole	Otomax	10 mg/g with gentamicin, betamethasone	Ointment	Schering-Plough	1
Clotrimazole	Lotrimin AF	2%	Topical spray	Schering-Plough	3

Generic Name	Proprietary Name	Strength	Form	Source	Approval
Clotrimazole	Lotrimin AF	1%	Lotion, topical	Schering-Plough	3
Clotrimazole	Lotrimin AF	2%	Topical spray powder	Schering-Plough	3
Clotrimazole	Lotrimin AF	20 mg/g	Topical powder	Schering-Plough	3
Clotrimazole	Gyne-Lotrimin 3	1%	Cream, vaginal	Schering-Plough	3
Clotrimazole	Gyne-Lotrimin 3	200 mg	Tablet, vaginal	Schering-Plough	3
Clotrimazole	Gyne-Lotrimin combo pack	1%, 100 mg	Cream, tablet, topical, vaginal	Schering-Plough	3
Clotrimazole	Gyne-Lotrimin combo pack	1% 200 mg	Cream, tablet, topical, vaginal	Schering-Plough	3
Cloxacillin	Cloxapen	250, 500 mg	Capsule	SmithKline Beecham	3
Cloxacillin	Orbenin-DC/Dari-Clox	500 mg in oil	10 mL syringe for intra-mammary infusion	Pfizer	4
Cloxacillin		125 mg/5 mL in 100 mL and 200 mL bottles	Oral solution		3
Codeine/acetaminophen	Codeine/acetaminoephen	12 mg/5 mL, 30 mg, 60 mg	Oral solution, capsule	Multiple	3
Codeine	Codeine phosphate, generic	15 mg, 30 mg, 60 mg	Tablet	Multiple	3
Coenzyme Q10 (ubiquinone)	Coenzyme Q	10 mg, 30 mg, 50 mg, 60 mg, 100 mg, 150 mg	Capsule	Multiple	D
Colchicine	Col-Bemeid, generic	0.5, 0.6	Tablet	Abbott, others	3

Generic Name	Proprietary Name	Strength	Form	Source	Approval
Colony-stimulating factor	Neupogen, see Filgrastin				
Cortisone acetate	Cortisone acetate	5 mg, 10 mg, 25 mg, 50 mg	Tablet	Pharmacia and Upjohn	3
Cortisone acetate	Cortone	25 mg/mL, 50 mg/mL	Injectable	Merck	3
Cortisone acetate	Cortone	25 mg	Tablet	Merck	3
Corticotropin	ACTH	25 Units/vial, 40 Units/vial	Injectable	Parke-Davis	3
Cosyntropin	Cortrosyn	250 μg vial	Injectable	Sandoz	
Cromolyn sodium 4%	Opticrom	4%	Opthalmic solution	Allergen	3
Cromolyn sodium	Intal	0.8 mg/puff	Metered aerosol	King Pharmaceuticals	3
Cromolyn sodium	Gastrocrom	100 mg/5 mL	Oral solution	UCB	3
Cromolyn sodium	Intal	10 mg/mL	Inhalation solution	King Pharmaceuticals	3
Cyanocobalamin (Vitamin B12)	Cyanocobalamin/vibisone	0.1 mg/mL, 1 mg/mL	Injectable	AM Pharm Partners	3
Cyanocobalamin	Nascobal	0.5 mg/puff	Metered nasal gel	Questcor	3
Cyclizine	Marezine	50 mg	Tablet	Himmel Pharmaceuticals	3, OTC
Cyclophosphamide	Lypholized cytoxan	75 mg mannitol/100 mg cyclophosphamide and 82 mg sodium	Injectable	Mead Johnson Oncology	3

Generic Name	Proprietary Name	Strength	Form	Source	Approval
continued—		bicarbonate/100 mg cyclopho-sphamide in 0.1 g, 0.2 g, 0.5 g, 1 g, 2 g vials			
Cyclophosphamide	Cytoxan	25 mg, 50 mg	Tablet	Mead Johnson Oncology	3
Cyclosporine	Sandimmune	50 mg/mL	Injectable	Novartis	3
Cyclosporine	Sandimmune	100 mg/mL	Oral solution	Novartis	3
Cyclosporine ophthalmic	Optimmune	0.20%	Opthalmic ointment	Schering-Plough	1
Cyclosporine	NeOral	25 mg, 50 mg, 100 mg	Capsule	Novartis	3
Cyclosporine	NeOral	100 mg/mL	Solution	Novartis	3
Cyproheptadine hydrochloride	Periactin	2 mg/5 mL	Syrup, oral	Merck	3
Cyproheptadine hydrochloride	Periactin	4 mg	Tablet	Merck	3
Cytarabine	Cytosar	100 mg vial	Injectable	Multiple	3
Cyothioate	Proban	30 mg	Tablet	Boehringer Ingelheim	1
Cytosine arabinoside	Cytosar-U	0.1 g/vial, 0.5 g/vial, 1 g/vial, 2 g/vial	Injectable	Pharmacia and Upjohn	3
Dacarbazine	DTIC-Dome	10 mg/mL in 10 mL and 20 mL vials	Injectable	Bayer	3

Generic Name	Proprietary Name	Strength	Form	Source	Approval
Dactinomycin	Cosmegen	0.5 mg in vials	Injectable lyophilized	Merck	3
Dalteparin	Fragmin	2500 IU, 5000 IU in 0.2 mL single dose syringes, 10,000 IU/mL in 9.5 mL multidose vials	Injectable	Eisai	3
Danazol	Danocrine	50 mg, 100 mg, 200 mg	Capsule	Sanofi-Synthelabo	3
Dantrolene	Dantrium	25 mg, 50 mg, 100 mg	Capsule	Procter and Gamble	3
Dantrolene	Dantrium	25 mg, 100 mg	Tablet, scored	Jacobus	3
Dapsone	Dapsone, generic	25 mg, 100 mg	Tablet	Multiple	3
Decoquinate	Deccox	0.5% (2271 mg/lb), 0.8% (3632 mg/lb), 6% (27.2 g/lb) feed additive	Feed additive (5 and 50 lb bags)	Alpharma	4
Deferoxamine mesylate	Desferal	500 mg vials	Injectable	Ciba	3
Demeclocycline	Declomycin	150 mg, 300 mg	Tablet	ESP Pharma	3
Deprenyl	Anipryl	2 mg, 5 mg, 10 mg, 15 mg, 30 mg	Tablet	Pfizer	1
Deprenyl	Eldipryl	5 mg	Tablet	Multiple	3
Deracoxib	Deramaxx	25 mg, 100 mg	Tablet	Novartis	1
Desmopressin acetate	DDAVP	0.01 mg/spray	Metered nasal spray	Aventis Pharmaceuticals	3

Generic Name	Proprietary Name	Strength	Form	Source	Approval
Desmopressin acetate	DDAVP	0.004 mg/mL, 0.015 mg/mL	Injectable	Aventis Pharmaceuticals	3
Desmopressin acetate	DDAVP	0.01%	Nasal solution	Aventis Pharmaceuticals	3
Desmopressin acetate	DDAVP	0.1 mg, 0.2 mg	Tablet	Aventis Pharmaceuticals	3
Desoxycorticosterone pivalate	Percorten-V	25 mg/mL	Injectable	Novartis	1
Dexamethasone	Azium, generic	0.25 mg, 0.5 mg, 0.75 mg, 1 mg, 1.5 mg, 2 mg, 4 mg, 6 mg	Tablet	Roxane, others	3
Dexamethasone	Azium solution	2 mg/mL	Injectable	Schering-Plough	1, 2
Dexamethasone sodium phosphate	Dexamethasone sodium phosphate	4 mg/mL	Injectable	Butler	4
Dexamethasone	Azium Solution	10 mg crystalline in 10 mg packets	Oral powder	Schering-Plough	4
Dexamethasone	Dexamethasone	0.5 mg/5 mL in 100 mL,120 mL, 240 mL, and 500 mL, 0.5 mg/mL in 30 mL with dropper	Oral solution	Roxane	3
Dexamethasone	Decadron	0.10%	Ophthalmic, otic solution	Merck	3
Dexpanthenol	D-panthenol	250 mg/mL in 100 mL vials	Injectable	Butler	1, 2, 4
Dexrazoxane	Zinecard	250 mg (25 mL vials), 500 mg (50 mL vials)	Injectable	Pharmacia	3
Dextran 40	Rheomacrodex	NI	NI	NI	3

Generic Name	Proprietary Name	Strength	Form	Source	Approval
Dextran 70	Macrodex	6% dextran 70 in 5% dextrose in 500 mL	Injectable	Medisan Pharmaceuticals	3
Dextroamphetamine	Dexedrine	5 mg	Tablet	GlaxoSmithKline	3
Dextroamphetamine	Dexedrine	5 mg, 10 mg, 15 mg	Capsule, extended release	GlaxoSmithKline	3
Dextrose 5%	D5W	5 g/100 mL	Injectable	Multiple	1, 2
Dextrose 50%	Cartose	50 g/mL	Injectable	Multiple	1, 2
Diazepam	Diazepam intensol	1 mg/mL in 500 mL and UD 5 and 10, 5 mg/mL in 30 mL with dropper, 5 mg/mL in 30, 500 mL UD 5	Oral solution	Roxane	3
Diazepam	Diastat	2.5 mg, 10 mg, 15 mg, 20 mg	Rectal gel	Elan	3
Diazepam	Valium, generic	2 mg, 5 mg, 10 mg	Tablet	Roche, others	3
Diazepam	Valium	5 mg/mL in 1 mL carton with syringes, 2 mL disposable syringes, 1 mL, 2 mL, 10 mL vials	Injectable	Roche	3
Diazoxide	Proglycem	50 mg	Capsule	Baker Norton	3
Diazoxide	Proglycem	50 mg/mL in 30 mL dropper bottles	Oral solution	Baker Norton	3
Diazoxide	Hyperstat	15 mg/mL in 20 mL ampules	Injectable	Schering-Plough	3
Dichlorphenamide	Daranide	50 mg	Tablet	Merck	3

Generic Name	Proprietary Name	Strength	Form	Source	Approval
Dichlorvos	Task	10 mg, 15 mg	Tablet	Boehringer Ingelheim	1, 2
Dicloxacillin	Dycill	125 mg, 250 mg, 500 mg	Capsule	GlaxoSmithKline	3
Dicloxacillin	Dynapen	12.5 mg/mL	Oral solution	Apothecon	3
Dicyclomine	Bentyl	10 mg/mL	Injectable	Axcan Scandipharm	3
Dicyclomine	Bentyl	10 mg	Capsule	Axcan Scandipharm	3
Dicyclomine	Bentyl	10 mg/5 mL	Syrup	Axcan Scandipharm	3
Dicyclomine	Bentyl	20 mg	Tablet	Axcan Scandipharm	3
Diethylcarbamazine	Hetrazan	50 mg	Tablet	Wyeth-Ayerst	3
Diethylcarbamazine	Nemacide, generic	Many	Tablet, chewable	Boehringer Ingelheim, others	1, 2
Diethystilbestrol	Stilphostrol	50 mg/mL	Injectable	Bayer	3
Difloxacin	Dicural	11.4 mg, 45.4 mg, 136 mg	Tablet, scored	Fort Dodge	1
Digoxin	Lanoxin	0.1 mg/mL, 0.25 mg/mL	Injectable	GlaxoSmithKline	3
Digoxin	Lanoxin	0.125 mg, 0.25 mg	Tablet	GlaxoSmithKline	3
Digoxin	Lanoxin	0.05 mg/mL	Oral solution	GlaxoSmithKline	3

Generic Name	Proprietary Name	Strength	Form	Source	Approval
Digoxin	Lanoxi-caps	0.05 mg, 0.1 mg, 0.2 mg	Capsule	GlaxoSmithKline	3
Dihydrotachysterol	Hytakerol	0.125 mg	Capsule	Sanofi Winthrop	3
Dihydrotachysterol	DHT	0.125 mg, 0.2 mg, 0.4 mg	Tablet	Roxane	3
Dihydrotachysterol	DHT Intensol	0.2 mg/mL in 30 mL dropper bottles	Oral solution	Roxane	3
Diltiazem	Cardizem CD	5 mg/mL in 5 mL, 10 mL, and 25 mL vials, 25 mg in single-use containers	Capsule, extended release	Biovail Pharmaceuticals	3
Diltiazem	Cardizem	30 mg, 60 mg, 90 mg, 120 mg	Capsule, extended release	Biovail Pharmaceuticals	3
Diltiazem XR, Cardiazem CD	Dilacor XR	60 mg, 90 mg, 120 mg, 180 mg, 240 mg, 300 mg, 360 mg, 420 mg	Capsule, extended release	Watson Labs	3
Dimenhydrinate	Dramamine	50 mg	Tablet	Upjohn	OTC
Dimenhydrinate	Dramamine	12.5 mg/4 mL in 90 mL, 12.5 mg/5 mL in 120 mL, 15.62 mg/5 mL in 480 mL	Oral liquid	Upjohn	OTC
Dimenhydrinate	Dinate	50 mg/mL	Injectable	Seatrace	3
Dimercaprol	BAL in oil	100 mg/mL (10%) in 3 mL ampules	Injectable IM	Taylor Pharmaceuticals	3
Dimethyl sulfoxide 40%	Domoso	90%	Topical liquid	Fort Dodge	1, 2

Generic Name	Proprietary Name	Strength	Form	Source	Approval
Dimethyl sulfoxide 50%	Rimso-50	50% aqueous solution in 50 mL	Aqueous solution	Research Industries	3
Diminazene aceturate	Berenil	NI	NI	NI	NI
Dioctyl sulfosuccinate	Surfak (Docusate)	NI	NI	NI	NI
Diphenhydramine hydrochloride	Benadryl	50 mg/mL	Injectable	Parke-Davis	3
Diphenhydramine hydrochloride	Benadryl, generic	12.5 mg, 25 mg, 50 mg	Capsule	Johnson and Johnson, others	3, OTC
Diphenhydramine hydrochloride	Benadryl, generic	12.5 mg/5 mL	Elixir	Johnson and Johnson, others	3, OTC
Diphenhydramine hydrochloride	Benadryl	2%	Topical spray	Warner Lambert	3
Diphenoxylate hydro-chlordie with atropine	Lomotil	0.05 mg/mL, 0.5 mg/mL	Oral solution	GD Searle LLC	3
Diphenoxylate hydro-chlordie with atropine	Lomotil	0.025 mg, 2.5 mg	Tablet	GD Searle LLC	3
Diphenylhydantoin	Dilantin-125	125 mg/5 mL	Oral suspension	Parke-Davis	3
Diphenylhydantoin	Dilantin	50 mg	Tablet, chewable	Pfizer	3
Diphenylhydantoin	Dilantin	30 mg, 100 mg extended	Capsule	Parke-Davis	3
Diphenylhydantoin	Phenytoin sodium	50 mg/mL	Injectable	Hospira	3
Dipyridamole with aspirin	Aggrenox	200 mg/25 mg	Capsule, extended release	Boehringer Ingelheim	3

Generic Name	Proprietary Name	Strength	Form	Source	Approval
Dipyridamole	Dipyridamole	5 mg/mL	Injectable	Baxter Healthcare	3
Dipyridamole	Persantine	25 mg, 50 mg, 75 mg	Tablet	Boehringer Ingelheim	3
Dipyrone	Novin	NI	NI	NI	
Dirlotapide	Slentrol	5 mg/mL	Oral suspension	Pfizer	1
Disodium EDTA	Disotate	NI	NI	NI	
Disopyramide PO_4	Norpace/Norpace CR	EQ 100 mg base, 150 mg base	Capsule, regular and extended release	Pharmacia	3
Dithiazanine iodide	Dizan	10 mg/tsp, 50 mg/tsp, 100 mg/tsp, 200 mg/tsp	Tablet, powder	Boehringer Ingelheim	1
Divalproex sodium	See Valproic acid	125 mg, 250 mg, 500 mg	Tablet, delayed release	Abbott	3
DL Methionine	Methio-Form, others	500 mg	Tablet		D
DL Methionine	NA	200 mg	Capsule		D
DL Methionine	NA	75 mg/mL	Oral solution		D
Dobutamine hydrochloride	Dobutrex	12.5 mg/mL in 20 mL vials	Injectable	Lilly	3
Docusate calcium	Surfak Liquigels	240 mg	Capsule	Pharmacia and Upjohn	OTC
Docusate sodium	Colace	50 mg, 100 mg, 240 mg,	Capsule	Roberts	OTC

Generic Name	Proprietary Name	Strength	Form	Source	Approval
Docusate sodium	Ex-lax Stool Softener	100 mg	Tablet	Novartis	OTC
Docusate sodium	Colace	20 mg/5 mL, 50 mg/15 mL, 60 mg/15 mL, 100 mg/30 mL	Syrup	Roberts	OTC
Docusate sodium	Colace	150 mg/15 mL in 30 mL and 480 mL	Liquid	Roberts	OTC
Docusate sodium	Bloat Release	240 mg/1 fl oz in 12 fl oz containers	Liquid	Agrilabs	OTC
Docusate sodium	Dioctynate	5% water miscible solution in 1 gal containers	Enema	Butler	OTC
Docusate sodium	Enema-DSS	250 mg in 12 mL syringes	Enema	Butler	OTC
Docusate sodium	Therevac-SB	283 mg	Gelatin ampules (soap base)	JPI Jones	OTC, 1, 2
Docusate sodium		5% in gallons	Oral liquid	Mutiple	OTC
Dolasetron mesylate		50 mg, 100 mg	Tablet	Aventis Pharmaceuticals	3
Dolasetron mesylate	Anzemet	20 mg/mL	Injectable	Aventis Pharmaceuticals	3
Dopamine hydrochloride	Inotropin	40 mg/mL, 80 mg/mL, 160 mg/mL in 5 mL ampules, 5 mL, 10 mL, 20 mL vials, 5 mL, 10 mL syringes	Injectable	Faulding	3
Dopamine hydrochloride in 5% dextrose for infusion		0.8 mg/mL, 1.6 mg/mL, 3.2 mg/mL in 250 and 500 mL	Injectable	Abbott	3

Generic Name	Proprietary Name	Strength	Form	Source	Approval
Doramectin	Dectomax	10 mg/mL	Injectable	Pfizer	4
Doxapram	Dopram-V	20 mg/mL in 20 mL multidose vials	Injectable	Fort Dodge	1, 2, 4
Doxepin hydrochloride	Sinequan	EQ 10 mg, 25 mg, 50 mg, 75 mg, 100 mg, 150 mg base	Capsule	Roerig	3
Doxorubicin hydrochloride	Adriamycin PFS	2mg/mL in 5, 10, 20, 25, 37.5 single dose vials and 100 mL multidose vials	Injectable	Pfizer	3
Doxorubicin hydrochloride	Doxil	20 mg in 10 mL vials	Injectable	Sequus	3
Doxycycline hydrochloride	Doxirobe	8.5% activity once mixed	Gel	Pfizer	1
Doxycycline (hyclate)	Vibramycin, generic	20 mg, 50 mg, 100 mg	Tablet and capsule	Pfizer, others	3
Doxycycline (monohydrate)	Monodox	50 mg, 75 mg, 100 mg	Tablet and capsule	Oclassen	3
Doxycycline (hyclate)	Doryx	75 mg and 100 mg	Coated pellets	Warner Chilcott	3
Doxycycline (monohydrate)	Vibramycin	5 mg/mL in 60 mL bottles	Powder for oral suspension	Pfizer	3
Doxycycline (calcium salt)	Vibramycin	10 mg/mL in 473 mL	Oral syrup	Pfizer	3
Doxycycline (hyclate 10%)	Atridox	42.5 mg in 2 syringe mixing system and blunt cannula	Injectable	CollaGenex	3

Generic Name	Proprietary Name	Strength	Form	Source	Approval
Doxycycline (hyclate)	Doxy 100 and 200	100 mg and 200 mg vials	Powder for injection	AAP	3
Doxylamine succinate	AH Tablets	25 mg, 100 mg	Tablet	Schering-Plough Animal Health	1
Doxylamine succinate	AH Injection	11.36 mg/mL	Injectable	Schering-Plough Animal Health	1
D-Penicillamine	See Penicillamine				
Edetate calcium disodium (calcium EDTA)	Calcium Disodium Versenate	200 mg/mL in 5 mL ampules (1 g/ampule)	Injectable	3M	3
Edrophonium chloride	Tensilon	10 mg/mL in 1 mL ampules and 10 mg/mL in 15 mL vials	Injectable	ICN	3
Edrophonium chloride (with atropine sulfate)	Enlon-Plus	10 mg/mL (with 0.14 mg/mL atropine sulfate) in 5 mL ampules and 15 mL multidose vials	Injectable	Ohmeda	3
Emodepside/praziquantel	Profender	0.35 mL, 0.7 mL, 1.12 mL	Topical	Bayer	2
Enalapril	Enacard	1 mg, 2.5 mg, 5 mg, 10 mg, 20 mg	Tablet	Merial	1
Enalapril	Vasotec	2.5 mg, 5 mg, 10 mg, 20 mg	Tablet	Biovail	3
Enalapril	Vasotec	1.25 mg/mL in 1 and 2 mL vials and 1 mL carpuject vials	Injectable IV	Biovail	3
Enflurane	Ethrane	99.90%	Inhalant	Baxter Healthcare	3
Enilconazole	Clinafarm EC	NI	Injectable	Schering-Plough Animal Health	4

Generic Name	Proprietary Name	Strength	Form	Source	Approval
Enoxaparin	Lovenox	100 mg/mL in 0.3 mL, 0.4 mL, 0.6 mL, 0.8 mL, 1 mL pre-filled syringes, 3 mL multidose vials	Injectable	Aventis Pharmaceuticals	3
Enrofloxacin	Baytril	22.7 mg, 68 mg, 136 mg	Tablet or taste tablet	Bayer	1, 2
Enrofloxacin	Baytril	22.7 mg/mL (2.27%) in 20 mL vials	Injectable	Bayer	1
Enrofloxacin	Baytril	3.23% (32.3 mg/mL)	Concentrate antimicrobial solution	Bayer	4, 5
Enrofloxacin	Baytril 100	100 mg/mL in 100 mL and 250 mL bottles	Injectable	Bayer	4
Ephedrine	Ephedrine Sulfate	25 mg	Capsule	West-Ward	OTC
Ephedrine	Ephedrine Sulfate	50 mg/mL in 1 mL ampules and vials	Injectable	Abbott	3
Epinephrine	Amtech Epinephrine Injection USP, generic	1 mg/mL (1:1,000) in 1 mL ampules and syringes and 10 mL, 30 mL, 100 mL vials	Injectable	Phoenix Scientific, others	1, 2, 3, 4
Epinephrine	Epi-pen	1 mg/mL (1:1,000) in 0.3 mL, 1 mL ampules, 5 mL vials, 1 mL tubex, 2 mL syringe, 30 mL sterile vials	Injectable	Dey	3
Epinephrine	Epi-pen Jr	0.5 mg/mL (1:2,000) in 0.3 mL single dose auto-injectors	Injectable	Dey	3
Epinephrine	Epinephrine	0.1 mg/mL (1:10,000) in 10 mL syringes, vials	Injectable	Abbott	3
Epoetin	Epogen	2,000 Units/mL	Injectable	Amgen	3

Generic Name	Proprietary Name	Strength	Form	Source	Approval
continued—		3,000 Units/mL, 4,000 Units/mL, 10,000 Units/mL, 20,000 Units/mL, 40,000 Units/mL in 1 mL and 2 mL vials			
Epsiprantel	Cestex	12.5 mg, 25 mg, 50 mg, 100 mg	Tablet, film coated	Pfizer	1, 2
Ergocalciferol (Vitamin D$_2$)	Drisdol	50,000 IU	Capsule	Sanofi-Synthelabo	3
Erythromycin	Gallimycin	100 mg/mL for IM injection (with 2% butylaminobenzoate as a local anesthetic) in 100 mL vials	Injectable	Bimeda	4, OTC
Erythromycin	Gallimycin Injection	200 mg/mL for IM injection in 100 mL, 250 mL, 500 mL vials	Injectable IM	Bimeda	4, OTC
Erythromycin	Gallimycin Dry Cow	50 mg/mL in 12 mL tubes	Injectable	AgriLabs	4, OTC
Erythromycin	Gallimycin - 36	300 mg/6 mL syringe	Mastitis infusion tube	Bimeda	4
Erythromycin	Ery-Tab, generic	250 mg, 333 mg, and 500 mg	Tablet, enteric coated	Abbott, others	3
Erythromycin	Erythromycin Filmtabs	250 mg, 500 mg	Tablet, film coated	Abbott	3
Erythromycin	PCE Dispertab	333 mg, 500 mg	Tablet with polymer coated particles	Abbott	3
Erythromycin	Eryc	250 mg	Capsule, extended release	Warner Chilcott	3
Erythromycin estolate	Ilosone	125 mg/5 mL, 250 mg/5 mL in 480 mL bottles	Oral suspension	Alpharma	3

Generic Name	Proprietary Name	Strength	Form	Source	Approval
Erythromycin stearate	Erythromycin Stearate	250 mg, 500 mg	Tablet, film coated	Abbott	3
Erythromycin ethylsuccinate	EES 400	400 mg	Tablet	Abbott	3
Erythromycin ethylsuccinate	EES Granules	200 mg/5 mL when reconstituted in 60 mL, 100 mL, 200 mL and UD 5 mL	Powder for oral suspension	Abbott	3
Erythromycin ethylsuccinate	EES 200	200 mg/5 mL in 100 mL, 480 mL	Oral suspension	Abbott	3
Erythromycin ethylsuccinate	EES 400	400 mg/5 mL in 100 mL and 480 mL	Oral suspension	Abbott	
Erythromycin	Ilotycin	0.50%	Ophthalmic ointment	Dista	3
Erythromycin ethylsuccinate	EryPed Drops	100 mg/2.5 mL in 50 mL	Oral suspension	Abbott	3
Erythromycin lactobionate	Eythrocin	500 mg and 1 g (as lactobionate) in vials	Injectable	Abbott	3
Erythromycin glucceptate	Ilotycin Glucceptate	1 g erythromycin (as glucceptate)/vial in 30 mL vials	Injectable	Lilly	3
Erythropoietin (human recombinant)	Epoetin alpha	2,000 Units/mL, 3,000 Units/mL, 4,000 Units/mL, 10,000 Units/mL, 20,000 Units/mL, 40,000 Units/mL in 1 and 2 mL vials	Injectable	Amgen	3, B
Esmolol	Brevibloc	10 mg/mL in 10 mL vials and 250 mg/mL in 10 mL ampules	Injectable	Baxter Healthcare	3

Generic Name	Proprietary Name	Strength	Form	Source	Approval
Essential fatty acids	DermCap	NI	NI	NI	D
Essential fatty acids	EFAVet-20	NI	NI	NI	D
Estradiol	Gynodiol	25.7 mg, 43.9 mg coated with not less than 0.5 mg oxytetracycline powder as a local anti-bacterial	Implants, controlled release	Vetlife	4
Estradiol cypionate	ECP	2 mg/mL in 50 mL vials	Injectable	Pharmacia	4
Estradiol cypionate	Depo-Estradiol	5 mg/mL in 5 mL vials	Injectable	Pharmacia	3
Estradiol	Estrace	0.5 mg, 1 mg, 1.5 mg, 2 mg	Tablet	Warner Chilcott	3
Ethacrynic acid	Edecrin	25 mg, 50 mg	Tablet	Merck	3
Ethacrynic acid) (ethacrynate sodium	Edecrin Sodium	50 mg ethacrynic sodium/ 50 mL vial after reconstitution	Injectable	Merck	3
Ethambutol	Myambutol	100 mg, 400 mg	Tablet	West-Ward	3
Ethanol 20%	Thunderbird	5% and 10% alcohol and 5% dextrose in water	Infusion	McGaw	3
Ethosuximide	Zarontin	250 mg	Capsule	Pfizer	3
Etidronate disodium	Didronel	200 mg, 400 mg	Tablet	Procter and Gamble Pharmaceuticals	3
Etidronate disodium	Didronel IV	50 mg/mL in 6 mL ampules (300 mg/ampule)	Injectable, IV infusion only	MGI Pharma	3

Generic Name	Proprietary Name	Strength	Form	Source	Approval
Etodolac	Etogesic	150 mg, 300 mg	Tablet, scored	Fort Dodge	1
Etodolac	Lodine	200 mg, 300 mg, 400 mg, 500 mg	Tablet and capsule	Wyeth-Ayerst	3
Etodolac	Lodine XL	400 mg, 500 mg, 600 mg	Tablet, extended release	Wyeth-Ayerst	3
Etomidate	Amidate	2 mg/mL in 10 mL, 20 mL ampules, single use vials, 20 mL Abboject syringes	Injectable	Hospira	3
Etretinate	Soriatane	10 mg, 25 mg	Capsule	Roche	3
Euthanasia solution (pentobarbital sodium)	Beuthanasia-D-Special	390 mg/mL/phenytoin sodium 50 mg/mL	Injectable	Schering-Plough	1
Euthanasia solution (pentobarbital sodium)	Fatal-Plus Powder	392 mg/mL when constituted to 250 mL with water	Injectable	Vortech	1, 2, 4
Euthanasia solution (pentobarbital sodium)	Sleepaway	260 mg/mL in 100 mL bottles (26%)	Injectable	Fort Dodge	1, 2
Euthanasia solution (pentobarbital sodium)	Socumb-6 gr	389 mg/mL in 100 mL and 250 mL vials	Injectable	Butler	1, 2
Euthanasia solution (pentobarbital sodium)	Fatal-Plus Solution	390 mg/mL in 250 mL vials	Injectable	Vortech	1, 2
Famotidine	Pepcid AC	10 mg (OTC), 20 mg, 40 mg	Tablet, gelcaps, and disintegrating tablet	Merck	3
Famotidine	Pepcic RPD	40 mg/5 mL in 400 mg bottles	Oral suspension	Merck	3

Generic Name	Proprietary Name	Strength	Form	Source	Approval
Famotidine	Pepcid	10 mg/mL in 1 mL and 2 mL single dose vials, 4 mL, 20 mL, 50 mL multidose vials, 20 mg/50 mL premixed in 50 mL single-dose container	Injectable	Merck	3
Febantel	Rintal, Vercom	27.2 mg, 163.3 mg	Tablet	Bayer	1, 2
Febantel	Rintal	9.30%	Oral suspension	Bayer	4
Felbamate	Felbatol	120 mg/mL in 240 mL and 960 mL bottles	Oral suspension	Wallace Labs	3
Felbamate	Felbatol	400 mg, 600 mg	Tablet	Wallace Labs	3
Fenbendazole	Panacur Granules 22.2%	222 mg/g (22.2%) in 0.18 oz, 1 g, 2 g, 4 g packets, 1 lb jars	Granule	Intervet	1
Fenbendazole	Panacur Granules 22.2%	222 mg/g (22.2%)	Granule	Intervet	4, OTC
Fenbendazole	Panacur Suspension	100 mg/mL (10%)	Oral suspension	Intervet	4, OTC
Fenbendazole	Panacur Paste	100 mg/mL (10%)	Oral suspension	Intervet	4, OTC
Fenbendazole	Safe-Guard Sweetlix	750 mg/lb in 25 lb block	Block	Intervet	4, OTC
Fenbendazole	Safe-Guard 0.96% Scoop Dewormer	1%	Type B medicated feed	Intervet	4, OTC
Fenbendazole	Safe-Guard Free-choice Cattle Dewormer	0.50% (2.27 g/lb)	Type C medicated feed	Intervet	4, OTC

Generic Name	Proprietary Name	Strength	Form	Source	Approval
Fenbendazole	Safe-Guard 0.5% Cattle Top Dress	1%	Pellets	Intervet	4, OTC
Fenbendazole	Safe-Guard 1.96% Scoop Dewormer Mini Pellets	2%	Pellets	Intervet	4, OTC
Fenbendazole	Safe-Guard Premix	20%	Type A premix	Intervet	4, OTC
Fentanyl citrate	Sublimaze, generic	250 mg/5 mL	Injectable	Multiple	1, 2, 3
Fentanyl	Sublimaze	0.05 mg/mL in 2 mL, 5 mL, 10 mL, 20 mL ampules	Injectable	Taylor Pharmaceuticals	3
Fentanyl	Duragesic- 25, 50, 75, 100	2.5 mg (25 μg/hr), 5 mg (50 μg/hr), 7.5 mg (75 μg/hr), 10 mg (100 μg/hr)	Extended release transdermal	Janssen	3
Fentanyl	Actiq	200 μg, 400 μg, 600 μg, 800 μg, 1200 μg, 1,600 μg	Transmucosal system (lozenges on a stick)	Abbott	3
Fenthion	Spotton	0.4 mg/mL fentanyl with 20 mg/mL droperidol	Injectable	Schering-Plough Animal Health	1
Ferrous sulfate	Feosol	324 mg (65 mg iron), 325 mg (65 mg iron) (20% elemental iron)	Tablet		OTC
Ferrous sulfate	Fer-In-Sol	90 mg/5 mL (18 mg iron/5 mL), 220 mg/5 mL (44 mg iron/5 mL) in 473 mL and 480 mL	Syrup	Mead Johnson Nutrition	OTC
Ferrous sulfate	Feosol	220 mg (44 mg iron)/ 5 mL in 473 mL	Elixir	SmithKline Beecham	OTC
Ferrous sulfate	Fer-In-Sol	75 mg/0.6 mL (15 mg iron /0.6 mL) in 50 mL	Drops	Mead Johnson Nutrition	OTC

Generic Name	Proprietary Name	Strength	Form	Source	Approval
Ferrous sulfate	Feosol	187 mg (60 mg iron), 200 mg (65 mg iron)	Tablet, dried (desiccated)	SmithKline Beecham	OTC
Ferrous sulfate	Slow FE	160 mg (50 mg iron)	Slow release tablet, dried (desiccated)	Novartis	OTC
Filgrastim	Neupogen	300 μg/mL in 1 mL, 1.6 mL single dose vials	Injectable	Amgen	3
Filgrastim	Neupogen	300 μg/0.5 mL in 0.5, 0.8 syringes		Amgen	3
Finasteride	Propecia	1 mg, 5 mg	Tablet	Merck	3
Fipronil	Frontline Topspot-Dog	0.67 mL, 1.34 mL, 2.68 mL, 4.02 mL	Topical solution	Merial	1, 2
Fipronil	Frontline Topspot-Cat	0.05 mL	Topical solution	Merial	1, 2
Fipronil with methoprene	Frontline Plus-Dog	0.67 mL, 1.34 mL, 2.68 mL, 4.02 mL	Topical solution	Merial	1, 2
Fipronil with methoprene	Frontline Plus-Cat	0.05 mL	Topical solution	Merial	1, 2
Firocoxib	Previcox	57 mg, 227 mg	Tablet	Merial	1
Flavoxate hydrochloride	Urispas	100 mg	Tablet	Ortho-McNeil Pharmaceuticals	3
Florfenicol	Nuflor	300 mg/mL in 100 mL, 250 mL, 500 mL multidose vials	Injectable	Schering-Plough Animal Health	4
Fluconazole	Diflucan in Dextrose 5% in plastic container	200 mg/100 mL	Injectable	Roerig	3

Generic Name	Proprietary Name	Strength	Form	Source	Approval
Fluconazole	Diflucan in Sodium Chloride 0.9%	200 mg/100 mL	Injectable	Roerig	3
Fluconazole	Diflucan in NaCl 0.9% in plastic container	200 mg/100 mL	Injectable	Roerig	3
Fluconazole	Diflucan	10 mg/mL (when reconstituted) in 350 mg, 40 mg/mL (when reconstituted) in 1400 mg	Powder for reconstitution, oral	Roerig	3
Fluconazole	Diflucan	50 mg, 100 mg, 150 mg, 200 mg	Tablet	Roerig	3
Flucytosine	Ancobon	250 mg, 500 mg	Capsule	ICN	3
Fludrocortisone	Florinef	0.1 mg	Tablet	Monarch Pharmacueticals	3
Flumazenil	Romazican	0.1 mg/mL in 5 mL, 10 mL vials	Injectable IV	Hoffman-LaRoche	3
Flumethasone	Flucort Solution	0.5 mg/mL in 100 mL vials	Injectable	Fort Dodge	1, 2, 4
Flunixin meglumine	Banamine	50 mg/mL in 50 mL, 100 mL, 250 mL vials	Injectable	Schering-Plough	4
Flunixin meglumine	Banamine Paste	1500 mg/syringe, 30 g syringe containing 1500 mg flunixin (in boxes of 6)	Oral paste	Schering-Plough	4
Flunixin meglumine	Banamine Granules	250 mg, 10 g sachets. Each sachet contains 250 mg flunixin (in boxes of 50)	Oral granule	Schering-Plough	4
Flunixin meglumine	Banamine Granules	500 mg, 20 g sachets. Each sachet contains 500 mg flunixin (in boxes of 25)	Oral granule	Schering-Plough	4

Generic Name	Proprietary Name	Strength	Form	Source	Approval
Fluorouracil	5-fluorouracil	50 mg/mL vial	Injectable	Multiple	3
5-Fluorouracil	Adrucil	50 mg/mL	Injectable	Sicor Pharmaceuticals, Pharmacia and Upjohn	3
Fluoxetine hydrochloride	Prozac Pulvules	10 mg, 20 mg, 40 mg, 90 mg (delayed release)	Capsule	Eli Lilly/Dista	3
Fluoxetine hydrochloride	Prozac	20 mg/5 mL in 120 mL, 473 mL	Oral solution	Eli Lilly/Dista	3
Fluoxetine hydrochloride	Prozac	10 mg, 20 mg	Tablet	Eli Lilly/Dista	3
Fluoxetine hydrochloride	Reconcile	8 mg, 16 mg, 32 mg, 64 mg	Tablet	Eli Lilly/Dista	1
Fluoxymesterone		2 mg, 5 mg, 10 mg	Tablet	Pharmacia and Upjohn	3
Flurazepam	Dalmane	15 mg, 30 mg	Capsule	Valeant Pharmaceuticals International	3
Flurbiprofen	Ocufen	0.03%	Ophthalmic solution	Allergan	3
Flurbiprofen	Ansaid	50 and 100 mg	Tablet	Pharmacia and Upjohn	3
Fluticosone proprionate	Flovent	1110, 220 mcg/actuation in 7.9 (60 metered inhalations) or 13 g (120 metered inhalations) canister	Inhalant device	GlaxoSmithKline	3
Fluvoxamine maleate	Luvox, generic	25, 50, 100 mg	Tablet	Jazz Pharmaceuticals	3
Folic acid	Folicet	1 mg	Tablet	Mission Pharma	3

Generic Name	Proprietary Name	Strength	Form	Source	Approval
Follicle-stimulating hormone	Super-OV	75 Units	Injectable	Ausa International Inc	4
Formoterol	Foradil	0.012 mg/inh	Inhalant, powder	Novartis	3
Formoterol	Perforomist	0.02 mg/2 mL	Inhalant, solution	Dey LP	3
Foscanart sodium	Foscavir	2.4 g/100 mL	Injectable	AstraZeneca	3
Furazolidone	Furoxone	100 mg	Tablet	Procter and Gamble	3
Furosemide	Lasix, generic	12.5 mg, 50 mg	Tablet	Intervet, others	1, 2
Furosemide	Lasix Injection 5%, generic	50 mg/mL (5%) in 50 mL, 100 mL vials	Injectable	Intervet, others	1, 2, 4
Furosemide	Lasix	20 mg, 40 mg, 80 mg	Tablet	Aventis Pharmaceuticals	3
Furosemide	Furosemide	10 mg/mL in 60 mL, 120 mL bottles, 40 mg/5 mL in 500 mL and UD 5 and 10 mL	Oral solution	Roxane	3
Furosemide	Furosemide	10 mg/mL in 10 mL, 2 mL, 4 mL, 10 mL single dose vials	Injectable	Roxane	3
Furosemide	Furosemide	20 mg, 40 mg, 80 mg	Tablet	Teva	3
Gabapentin	Neurontin	100 mg, 300 mg, 400 mg	Capsule	Pfizer	3
Gabapentin	Neurontin	50 mg/mL in pint bottles	Oral solution	Pfizer	3

Generic Name	Proprietary Name	Strength	Form	Source	Approval
Gabapentin	Neurontin	600 mg, 800 mg	Tablet, film coated	Pfizer	3
Gamma globulin	Gamma globulin	NI	NI	NI	B
Gemfibrozil	Lopid, generic	600 mg	Tablet	Pfizer	3
Gentamicin sulfate 0.1%	Gentocin	50 mg/mL, 100 mg/mL (horses only) in 50 mL, 100 mL, 250 mL vials	Injectable	Schering-Plough	1, 2, 4
Gentamicin sulfate	Garacin Piglet Injection	5 mg/mL in 250 mL vials	Injectable	Schering-Plough	4
Gentamicin sulfate	Garacin Oral Solution	50 mg/mL in 80 mL bottles	Oral solution	Schering-Plough	4
Gentamicin sulfate	Gen-Guard Soluble Powder	333.33 mg/g in 18 g packets	Soluble powder	AgriLabs	4, OTC
Gentamicin sulfate	Garacin Pig Pump Oral Solution	4.35 mg/mL in 115 mL pump bottles (1 pump delivers approximately 5 mg)	Oral solution	Schering-Plough	4
Gentamicin sulfate	Garacin Soluble Powder	2 g gentamicin/30 g of powder in 360 g jar	Soluble powder	Schering-Plough Animal Health	4, OTC
Gentamicin sulfate	Gentocin Otic	3 mg/mL gentocin with betamethasone 1 mg/mL	Otic solution	Schering-Plough Animal Health	1, 2
Gentamicin sulfate	Gentocin Otic	0.57 mg/mL gentocin with 0.28 mg/mL betamethasone	Topical spray	Schering-Plough Animal Health	1

Generic Name	Proprietary Name	Strength	Form	Source	Approval
Gentamicin sulfate	Garamycin	40 mg/mL in 2 mL, 20 mL vials, 1.5 mL, 2 mL cartridge-needle Units, 10 mg/mL in 2 mL vials	Injectable	Schering-Plough Animal Health	3
Glipizide	Glucotrol XL	2.5, 5, 10 mg	Tablet, extended release	Pfizer	3
Glipizide	Glucotrol	5, 10mg	Tablet	Pfizer	3
Glucagon	Gluco-Gen	1 mg (1 unit) with 1 mL diluentin vials	Injectable	Bedford	3
Glucose 40% ophthalmic	Glucose-40	NI	NI	NI	NI
Glyburide		1.25 mg, 2.5 mg, 5 mg micronized tablets, 1.5 mg, 3 mg, 4.5 mg, 6 mg	Tablet	Pharmacia and Upjohn	3
Glyburide/metformin hydrochloride	Glucovance	1.25 mg/ 250 mg, 2.5 mg/500 mg, 5 mg/500 mg	Tablet	Bristol-Myers Squibb	3
Glycerin	Osmoglyn, others	50% (0.6 g glycerin/mL) in 220 mL	Oral liquid	Alcon, others	3
Glyceryl guaiacolate	Gecolate	50 mg/mL with 50 mg/mL glucose	Injectable	Summitt Hills	4
Glycerol monoacetate	Glycerol monoacetate	NI	NI	NI	NI
Glycopyrrolate	Robinul-V	0.2 mg/mL in 20 mL vials	Injectable Δ242	Fort Dodge	1, 2

Generic Name	Proprietary Name	Strength	Form	Source	Approval
Glycopyrrolate	Robinul	1 mg, 2 mg	Tablet	Horizon	3
Glycopyrrolate	Robinul	0.2 mg/mL in 1 mL, 2 mL, 5 mL, 20 mL vials	Injectable	Robins	3
Gold sodium thiomalate	Myochrysine	50 mg/mL	Injectable	Merck	3
Gonadotropin-releasing hormone (synthetic)	Gondorelin	50 μg/mL in 2 mL single use or 10 mL multidose vials	Injectable	Intervet	4
Gonadotropin-releasing hormone (synthetic)	Gonadorelin	50 μg/mL in 2 mL single use and 20 mL multidose vials	Injectable	Fort Dodge	4
Gonadotropin-releasing hormone (synthetic)	Gonadorelin	100 μg/vial, 500 μg/vial with 2 mL sterile diluent	Powder for injection (lyophilized)	Wyeth-Ayerst	3
Granisetron hydrochloride	Kytril	0.1 mg base/mL, 1 mg base/mL (EQ 1 mg base/mL), 4 mg base/ 4mL (EQ 1 mg base/mL)	Injectable	Apotex	3
Granisetron hydrochloride	Kytril	1.12 mg	Tablet	Apotex	3
Granisetron hydrochloride	Kytril	2 mg base/10 mL	Oral solution	Roche	3
Granisetron hydrochloride	Kytril	EQ 1 mg base	Tablet	Roche	3
Griseofulvin	Fulvicin	2.5 g griseofulvin in 15 g sachets	Powder (microsize)	Schering-Plough	4
Griseofulvin	Fulvicin-U/F Tablets	250 mg, 500 mg	Tablet (microsize)	Schering-Plough	1, 2
Griseofulvin	Gris-PEG	125 mg, 165 mg, 250 mg, 330 mg	Tablet (ultramicrosize)	Pedinol	3

Generic Name	Proprietary Name	Strength	Form	Source	Approval
Guaifenesin	Guailaxin	50 g for reconstitution in 4 oz, 32 oz containers	Injectable (powder)	Fort Dodge	4
Guaifenesin	Robitussin	NI	NI	NI	OTC
Guaifenesin	Guaifenesin Injection	50 mg/mL in 1000 mL	Injectable	Butler	4
Halothane	Fluothane	USP (with thymol 0.01% and ammonia 0.00025%) in 250 mL bottles	Inhalant	Halocarbon	1, 2, 4
Halothane	Halothane	250 mL bottles	Inhalant	Abbott	3
Hemoglobin	Polymerized bovine, Oxyglobin	60 mL and 250 mL ready to use infusion bags	IV infusion	Biopure	1
Heparin sodium	Heparin	1,000 Units/mL, 2,000 Units/mL, 2,500 Units/mL, 5,000 Units/mL, 10,000 Units/mL, 20,000 Units/mL, 40,000 Units/mL in 0.5 mL, 1 mL, 2 mL, 4 mL, 5 mL, 10 mL, 30 mL ampules and vials	Injectable	Various	3
Heparin sodium	Heparin Sodium	1,000 Units/dose, 2,000 Units/dose, 5,000 Units/dose, 7,500 Units/dose, 10,000 Units/dose, 20,000 Units/dose in 1 mL, 10 mL, 30 mL vials	Injectable	Elkins-Sinns	3
Heparin sodium (with 0.9% sodium chloride)		1,000 Units, 2,000 Units in 500 mL, 1000 mL Viaflex, respectively	Injectable	Baxter Healthcare	3

Generic Name	Proprietary Name	Strength	Form	Source	Approval
Heparin sodium (with 0.45% sodium chloride)		12,500 Units, 25,000 Units in 250 mL, 500 mL	Injectable	Abbott	3
Heparin sodium (lock flush solution)	Hep-Lock	10 Units/mL, 100 Units/mL in 1 mL, 2 mL, 5 mL, 10 mL, 30 mL, 50 mL vials	Injectable IV	Elkins-Sinn	3
Hetacillin	Hetacin-K	50 mg, 100mg, 200 mg	Tablet	Fort Dodge	1, 2
Hetacillin	Hetacin-K	50 mg/mL	Oral solution	Fort Dodge	1, 2
Hetastarch	Hetastarch	6% (6 g/100 mL) hetastarch in 0.9% NaCl in 500 mL IV infusion containers	Injectable	Gensia Sicor Pharmaceuticals	3
Hyaluronate (hyaluronan)	Hylalovet	20 mg/mL in 2 mL disposable syringes	Injectable	Fort Dodge	4
Hyaluronate (sodium)	Legend	2 mL vial for intraarticular administration, 4 mL vials for IV administration	Injectable	Pharmacia and UpJohn	4
Hyaluronate (sodium)	Hyvisc	11 mg/mL in 2 mL syringes	Injectable	Boehringer Ingelheim	4
Hyaluronate (sodium)	Hylartin	10 mg/mL in 2 mL disposable syringes	Injectable	Pfizer	4
Hyaluronate (sodium)	Hycoat	10 mg/mL	Injectable	Neogen	4
Hydralazine	Apresoline, generic	10 mg, 25 mg, 50 mg, 100 mg	Tablet	Multiple	1, 2, 3
Hydralazine	Apresoline, generic	20 mg/mL	Injectable	Multiple	1, 2, 3

Generic Name	Proprietary Name	Strength	Form	Source	Approval
Hydrochlorothiazide	HydroDiuril, generic	25 mg, 50 mg, 100 mg	Tablet	Merck, others	3
Hydrochlorothiazide (metoprolol tartrate)	Lopressor	12.5 mg	Capsule	Watson	3
Hydrochlorothiazide (spironolactone)	Aldactazide	10 mg/mL in 500 mL bottles	Oral solution	Roxane	3
Hydrocodone bitartrate	Hycodan	5 mg, homatropine MBr 1.5 mg	Tablet	Endo Pharms	3
Hydrocodone bitartrate	Hycodan Syrup	5 mg, homatropine MBr 1.5 mg (per 5 mL) in 473 mL and 3.8 L	Oral syrup	Endo Pharms	3
Hydrocortisone sodium succinate	Solu-Cortef	100 mg/vial, 250 mg/vial, 500 mg/vial, 1,000 mg/vial in 2 mL, 4 mL, 8 mL vials	Injectable	Upjohn	3
Hydrocortisone	Acticort 100, generic	1%	Topical lotion	Baker Norton, others	3
Hydrocortisone	Cortef, generic	5 mg, 10 mg, 20 mg	Tablet	Upjohn, others	3
Hydrocortisone acetate	Hydrocortone Acetate	25 mg/mL, 50 mg/mL in 5 mL and 10 mL vials	Injectable	MSD	3
Hydrocortisone cypionate	Cortef	2 mg/mL hydrocortisone in 120 mL	Oral suspension	Upjohn	3
Hydrocortisone sodium phosphate	Hydrocortone Phosphate	50 mg/mL solution in 2 mL and 10 mL vials	Injectable	MSD	3
Hydrogen peroxide 3%	Hydrogen peroxide 3%, generic	3%	Topical solution	Multiple	OTC

Generic Name	Proprietary Name	Strength	Form	Source	Approval
Hydromorphone	Dilaudid, generic	1 mg/mL, 2 mg/mL, 4 mg/mL, 10 mg/mL	Injectable IV	Abbott, others	3
Hydromorphone	Dilaudid-HP	250 mg (10 mg/mL after reconstitution) in single dose vials	Injectable (powder, lyophilized)	Abbott	3
Hydromorphone	Dilaudid	2 mg, 4 mg, 8 mg	Tablet	Abbott	3
Hydromorphone	Dilaudid-5	5 mg/5 mL in 120 mL, 250 mL, 473 mL, 500 mL	Oral liquid	Abbott	3
Hydromorphone	Dilaudid	3 mg	Rectal suppository	Abbott	3
Hydroxyethyl starch	Hetastarch	6% hetastarch in 0.9% NaCl	Injectable	Abbott, Baxter Healthcare	3, B
Hydroxyurea	Droxia	200 mg, 300 mg, 400 mg, 500 mg	Capsule	Bristol-Myers Squibb	3
Hydroxyurea	Mylocel	100 mg	Tablet	MGI Pharma	3
Hydroxyzine	Atarax	10 mg, 25 mg, 50 mg, 100 mg	Tablet	Roerig	3
Hydroxyzine	Atarax	10 mg/5 mL in 16 mL, 118 mL, 120 mL, 473 mL, gallons	Oral solution	Roerig	3
Hydroxyzine	Vistaril	25 mg/mL, 50 mg/mL	Injectable	Roerig	3
Hydroxyzine pamoate	Vistaril	25 mg, 50 mg, 100 mg	Capsule	Pfizer	3
Hydroxyzine pamoate	Vistaril	25 mg/5 mL in 120 mL, 473 mL, 480 mL	Oral suspension	Pfizer	3
Hypertonic saline	Hypertonic saline	NI	NI	NI	3

Generic Name	Proprietary Name	Strength	Form	Source	Approval
Idarubicin	Idamycin PFS	1 mg/mL	Injectable	Pharmacia and UpJohn	3
Idarubicin hydrochloride	Idarubicin hydrochloride	5 mg/mL, 10 mg/mL, 20 mg/mL	Injectable	Teva	3
Idarubicin hydrochloride	Idarubicin hydrochloride	1 mg/mL	Injectable	Pharmacia and UpJohn, Bedford	3
Ifosfamide (mesna)	IFEX/Mesnex Kit	1 g, 3 g for IV infusion in single dose vials (with mesna 100 mg/mL)	Injectable	Bristol-Myers Squibb	3
Imidocarb dipropionate	Imizol	120 mg/mL in 10 mL multidose vials	Injectable (IM or SC)	Schering-Plough Animal Health	1
Imidacloprid	Advantage	0.4 mL, 1 mL, 2.5 mL, 4 mL applicatiors	Topical solution	Bayer	1
Imidacloprid/moxidectin	Advantage Multi-Dogs	0.4 mL, 1 mL, 2.5 mL, 4 mL applicatiors	Topical solution	Bayer	1
Imidacloprid/moxidectin	Advantage Multi-Cats	0.23 mL, 0.4 mL, 0.8 mL	Topical solution	Bayer	2
Imidacloprid/permethrin	Advantix	0.4 mL, 1 mL, 2.5 mL, 4 mL applicatiors	Topical	Bayer	1
Imipenem/cilastatin	Primaxin IV	250 mg, 250 mg cilastatin (0.8 mEq sodium), 500 mg, 500 mg cilastatin (1.6 mEq) sodium	Injectable	Merck	3
Imipenem/cilastatin	Primaxin IM	500 mg, 500 mg cilastatin (1.4 mEq sodium), 750 mg, 750 mg cilastatin (2.1 mEq sodium)	Injectable	Merck	3
Imipramine	Tofranil	10 mg, 25 mg, 50 mg	Tablet	Novartis	3
Imipramine	Tofranil-PM	75 mg, 100 mg, 125 mg	Capsule	Novartis	3
Insulin, regular	Vetsulin	40 Units/mL	Injectable	NI	1

Generic Name	Proprietary Name	Strength	Form	Source	Approval
Insulin, lente	NI	100 Units/mL	Injectable	NI	3
Insulin, NPH	NI	100 Units/mL	Injectable	NI	3
Insulin, PZI	PZI Insulin	40 Units/mL	Injectable	Blue Ridge Pharmacy	1, 2
Insulin, ultralente	NI	100 Units/mL	Injectable	NI	
Interferon α2	Roferon-A	3 IU, 6 IU, 9 IU, 18 IU, 36 IU/syringe, vial	Injectable	Hoffman La-Roche	3
Iohexol	Omnipaque 140	30.20%	Injectable	GE Healthcare	3
Iohexol	Omnipaque 350	75.50%	Solution, injectable, oral	GE Healthcare	3
Iohexol	Omnipaque 180	38.80%	Solution, injectable, oral, rectal	GE Healthcare	3
Iohexol	Omnipaque 240	51.80%	Solution, iinjectable, oral, rectal	GE Healthcare	3
Iohexol	Omnipaque 300	64.70%	Solution, injectable, oral, rectal	GE Healthcare	3
Iopamidol	Isovue-200	41%	Injectable	Bracco	3
Iopamidol	Isovue-250	51%	Injectable	Bracco	3
Iopamidol	Isovue-300	61%	Injectable	Bracco	3
Iopamidol	Isovue-370	76%	Injectable	Bracco	3

Generic Name	Proprietary Name	Strength	Form	Source	Approval
Iopamidol	Isovue-M 200	41%	Injectable	Bracco	3
Iopamidol	Isovue-M 300	61%	Injectable	Bracco	3
Ipecac syrup	NA	1.5%, 1.75% alchohol in 15 mL, 30 mL, 2% alcohol in 15 mL, 30 mL	Oral solution	Various	3, OTC
Isoflurane	Isoflo	99.90%	Inhalant	Abbott	1,4
Isoniazid	Isoniazid	10 mg/mL	Oral solution	Carolina Medical	3
Isoniazid	Isoniazid	100 mg/mL	Injectable	Sabex 2002	3
Isoniazid	Laniazid	50 mg, 100 mg, 300 mg	Tablet	Lannett	3
Isopropamide/ prochlorperazine	Darbazine	0.38/6 mg/mL	Injectable	Pfizer	1, 2
Isopropamide/ prochlorperazine	Darbazine	1.67 mg/3.33 mg	Tablet	Pfizer	1
Isoproterenol	Isuprel	0.2 mg/mL	Injectable	Sanofi Winthrop	3
Isosorbide dinitrate	Isordil	5 mg, 10 mg, 20 mg, 30 mg, 40 mg	Tablet	BioVail	3
Isosorbide dinitrate	Dilatrate-SR	40 mg	Capsule, extended release	Schwarz Pharm	3
Isosorbide dinitrate	Isordil	2.5 mg, 5 mg, 10 mg	Tablet, sublingual	BioVail	3

Generic Name	Proprietary Name	Strength	Form	Source	Approval
Isosorbide mononitrate	Isosorbide Mononitrate	30 mg, 60 mg, 120 mg	Tablet, extended release	Ivax Pharms	3
Isosorbide mononitrate	Monoket	10 mg, 20 mg	Tablet	Schwarz	3
Isotretinoin	Accutane	10 mg, 20 mg, 40 mg	Capsule	Roche	3
Isoxsuprine	Vasodilan	10 mg, 20 mg	Tablet	Mead Johnson	3
Itraconazole	Sporanox	100 mg	Capsule	Janssen	3
Itraconazole	Sporanox	10 mg/mL	Injectable	Ortho Biotech	3
Itraconazole	Sporanox	10 mg/mL	Oral solution	Janssen	3
Ivermectin	Heartgard-30	68, 136, 272 ivermectin/57, 114, 227 pyrantel mg/mL	Tablet, chewable cubes	Merial	1
Ivermectin/pyrantel	Heartgard-Plus	68 mg/mL, 136 mg/mL, 272 mg/mL	Tablet, chewable cubes	Merial	1
Ivermectin	Heartgard	55 mg, 165 mg	Tablet	Merial	2
Ivermectin	Ivomec	1%	Injectable	Merial	4
Ivermectin (with praziquantel)	Equimax	1.87% with 14.03% praziquantel	Oral syringes	Pfizer	4
Ivermectin	Ivomec Pour-on	5 mg/mL	Pour on topical	Merial	4

Generic Name	Proprietary Name	Strength	Form	Source	Approval
Kanamycin	Kantrex	75 mg base/2 mL, 500 mg base/2 mL, 1 g base/3 mL	Injectable	Apothecan	3
Kaolin/pectin	Kaopectate	750 mg attapulgite	Oral solution	Pharmacia and UpJohn	OTC
Kaolin/pectin	Kaolin Pectin Plus	90 g kaolin/2 g pectin per fl oz	Oral solution	Agripharm	1, 2, 4
Ketamine hydrochloride	Ketaset	100 mg/mL	Injectable	Fort Dodge	1
Ketamine hydrochloride	Ketalar	10 mg/mL, 50 mg/mL, 100 mg/mL	Injectable	Monarch Pharmaceuticals	3
Ketamine hydrochloride/ aminopentamide/ promazinepromazine	Ketaset-Plus	100/0.0625/7.5 mg/mL, respectively	Injectable	Fort Dodge	1
Ketoconazole	NizOral	200 mg	Tablet	Janssen	3
Ketoprofen	Orudis, generic	50 mg, 75 mg	Capsule	Andrx	3
Ketoprofen	Ketofen	100 mg/mL	Injectable	Fort Dodge	4
Ketoprofen	Orudis KT	12.5 mg	Tablet	Whitehall-Robins	3, OTC
Ketoprofen	Oruvail	100 mg, 150 mg, 200 mg	Capsule, extended release	Wyeth-Ayerst	3
Ketorolac tromethamine	Acular (PF)	0.50%	Ophthalmic solution	Allergan Optical	3
Ketorolac tromethamine	Toradol	15 mg/mL, 30 mg/mL	Injectable	Roche	3
Ketorolac tromethamine	Toradol	10 mg	Tablet	Roche	3

Generic Name	Proprietary Name	Strength	Form	Source	Approval
Lactated Ringer's Solution	LRS	250 mL, 500 mL, 1000 mL	Injectable		
Lactoferrin	Lactoferrin	NI	NI	NI	NI
Lactulose	Cephulac	10 g/15 mL	Oral syrup	Hoechst-Marion Roussel	3
Lactulose	Chronulac	0.75 mg/mL	Oral/rectal solution	Aventis Pharmaceuticals	3
L-Carnitine	Carnitor	200 mg/mL	Injectable	Sigma Tau	3
L-Carnitine	Carnitor	1 g/10 mL	Oral solution	Sigma Tau	3
L-Carnitine	Carnitor	330 mg	Tablet	Sigma Tau	3
Leucovorin	Wellcovorin	5 mg/mL, 100 mg/mL	Injectable	GlaxcoSmithKline	3
Leucovorin calcium	Leucovorin	5 mg, 10 mg, 15 mg, 25mg	Tablet	Multiple***	3
Leucovorin calcium	Leucovorin	10 mg/vial, 50 mg/vial, 100 mg/vial, 200 mg/vial, 350 mg/vial, 500 mg/vial	Injectable	Multiple***	3
Levamisole	Ergamisol	50 mg	Tablet	Janssen	3
Levamisole	Tramisol Injectable	136.5 mg/mL	Injectable	Schering-Plough	4
Levamisole	Tramisol Type A Medicated Article	50% (227 g/lb)	Feed medication	Schering-Plough	4, OTC

Generic Name	Proprietary Name	Strength	Form	Source	Approval
Levamisole	Totalon	200 mg/mL	Pour on topical	Schering-Plough	4, OTC
Levetiracetam	Keppra	250 mg, 400 mg, 750 mg	Tablet	UCB	3
Levetiracetam	Keppra	100 mg/mL (240 mL)	Oral solution	UCB	3
Levoamphetamine	Levo-amphetamine	NI	NI	NI	NI
Levodopa	Carbidopa and Levodopa	100 mg (with10 mg carbidopa), 100 mg (with 25 mg carbidopa), 250 mg (with 25 mg carbidopa)	Tablet	Teva	3
Levorphanol tartrate	Levo-Dromoran	2 mg/mL	Injectable	Valeant Pharmaceuticals International	3
Levorphanol tartrate	Levorphanol Tartrate	2 mg	Tablet	Roxane	3
Levothyroxine, T_4	Thyroxine-L tablets	0.1 mg, 0.2 mg, 0.3 mg, 0.4 mg, 0.5 mg, 0.6 mg, 0.7 mg, 0.8 mg	Tablet	Butler	1
Levothyroxine, T_4	Synthyroid	0.025 mg, 0.05 mg, 0.075 mg, 0.88 mg, 0.1 mg, 0.112 mg, 0.125 mg, 0.137 mg, 0.15 mg, 0.175 mg, 0.2 mg, 0.3 mg	Tablet	Abbott	3
Levothyroxine, T_4	Nutrived T-4 Chewable Tablets	0.1 mg, 0.2 mg, 0.3 mg, 0.4 mg, 0.5 mg, 0.6 mg, 0.7 mg, 0.8 mg	Tablet, chewable	Vedco	1
Levothyroxine, T_4	Throxine-L Powder	0.22% (1 g of T_4 in 454 g powder)	Powder	Butler	4
Lidocaine	Anestacon	2%	Topical	Polymedica	3

Generic Name	Proprietary Name	Strength	Form	Source	Approval
Lidocaine	Lidocaine	20%	Injectable	Hospira	3
Lidocaine	Xylocaine, generic	0.5%, 1%, 1.5%, 2%, 4%, 10%, 20% with or without epineprhine	Injectable	AstraZeneca, others	3
Lidocaine	Xylocaine Viscous	2%	Oral solution	AstraZeneca	3
Lidocaine	LTA Kit	2%, 4%	Topical solution	Hospira	3
Lime sulfur suspension	Sulfodip	NI	NI	NI	OTC
Lime water	Vlemasque	NI	NI	NI	NI
Lincomycin	Lincocin	100 mg, 200 mg, 500 mg	Tablet	Pharmacia and UpJohn	1, 2
Lincomycin	Lincocin Aquadrops	50 mg/mL	Oral solution	Pharmacia and Upjohn	1, 2
Lincomycin	Lincocin	100 mg/mL	Injectable	Pharmacia and Upjohn	1, 2
Linezolid	Zyvox	20 mg/mL	Oral suspension	Pharmacia and Upjohn	3
Linezolid	Zyvox	2 mg/mL	Injectable	Pharmacia and Upjohn	3
Linezolid	Zyvox	600 mg	Tablet	Pharmacia and Upjohn	3
Liothyronine, T_3	Cytomel	5 μg, 25 μg, 50 μg	Tablet	Monarch Pharmaceuticals	3
Liothyronine, T_3	Triostat	10 μg/mL	Injectable	Monarch Pharmaceuticals	3

Generic Name	Proprietary Name	Strength	Form	Source	Approval
Lisinopril	Prinivil	2.5 mg, 5 mg, 10 mg, 20 mg, 30 mg, 40mg	Tablet	Merck	3
Lithium carbonate	Lithium	150 mg, 300 mg, 600 mg	Capsule	Multiple	3
Lomustine	CeeNu	10 mg, 40 mg, 100 mg	Capsule	Bristol Labs Oncology	3
Loperamide hydrochloride	Imodium A-D	1 mg/5 mL	Oral solution	McNeil	3
Loperamide hydrochloride	Imodium A-D	2 mg	Tablet, chewable	McNeil	3
Loperamide hydrochloride	Imodium	2 mg	Capsule	Teva	3, OTC
Loperamide hydrochloride	Imodium A-D, generic	2 mg	Tablet	McNeil, others	3, OTC
Loperamide hydrochloride simethicone	Imodium Advanced	2 mg, 125 mg	Tablet, chewable	McNeil	3
Loratadine	Claratin, others	10 mg	Tablet	Multiple	3, OTC
Loratadine	Claratin, others	1 mg/mL	Oral syrup	Multiple	3, OTC
Lufenuron/milbemycin	Sentinel	46 mg, 115 mg, 230 mg, 460 mg (wtih nitenpyram)	Tablet	Novartis	1
Lufenuron	Program	45 mg, 90 mg, 204.9 mg, 409.8 mg (with nitenpyram)	Tablet	Novartis	1
Lufenuron	Program	90, 204.9 mg (with nitenpyram)	Tablet	Novartis	2
Lufenuron	Program	100 mg/mL	Injectable	Novartis	2

Generic Name	Proprietary Name	Strength	Form	Source	Approval
Lufenuron	Program Suspension	135 mg, 270 mg	Oral suspension	Novartis	2
Mafenide acetate	Sulfamylon cream	85 mg/g, 5%	Topical cream or solution	Bertek	3
Magnesium chloride	Generic	20% in 50 mL vials	Injectable	Hospira	3
Magnesium citrate	Evac-Q-Mag, Citroma	6%	Oral suspension	NA	OTC
Magnesium hydroxide	Milk of Magnesia, Mylanta	80 mg/mL	Oral solution	Multiple	OTC
Magnesium sulfate	Generic	10%, 12.5%, 50%	Injectable	QOL Medical	3
Mannitol 20%	Osmitrol	5%, 10%, 15%, 20%, 25% (50 mg/mL, 100 mg/mL, 150 mg/mL, 200 mg/mL, 250 mg/mL)	Injectable	Baxter Healthcare	3
Marbofloxacin	Zenoquin	25 mg, 50 mg, 100 mg, 200 mg	Tablet	Pfizer	1, 2
Maropitant	Cerenia	16 mg, 24 mg, 60 mg, 160 mg	Tablet	Pfizer	1
Maropitant	Cerenia	10 mg/mL	Injectable	Pfizer	1
Mebendazole	Telmintic	40 mg, 166.7 mg	Oral powder	Schering-Plough Animal Health	1
Meclizine	Dramamine Less Drowsy Formula	12.5 mg, 25 mg, 50 mg	Capsule or tablet	Multiple	OTC
Meclizine	Antivert	12.5 mg, 25 mg, 50 mg	Tablet	Pfizer	3

Generic Name	Proprietary Name	Strength	Form	Source	Approval
Meclofenamic acid	Meclofen, Arquel	50 mg, 100 mg	Capsule	Fort Dodge	NI
Meclofenamic acid	Meclofen, Arquel	10 mg, 20 mg	Tablet	Fort Dodge	NI
Medetomidine hydrochloride	Domitor	1 mg/mL	Injectable	Pfizer	1
Medium chain triglycerides	MCT in oil	NE	Oral	Mead Johnson Nutrition	OTC, 5
Medroxyprogesterone acetate	Depo-Provera	400 mg/mL	Injectable	Pharmacia and UpJohn	3
Medroxyprogesterone acetate	Provera, generic	2.5 mg, 5 mg, 10 mg	Tablet	Pharmacia and UpJohn, others	3
Megestrol acetate	Megace	40 mg/mL	Oral suspension	Bristol-Meyers Oncology	3
Megestrol acetate	Ovaban	5 mg, 20 mg	Tablet	Schering-Plough Animal Health	1
Megestrol acetate	Megace	20 mg, 40 mg	Tablet	Bristol-Meyers Oncology	3
Meglumine antimonate	Glucantime	NA	NA	NA	5
Melarsomine hydrochloride	Immiticide	25 mg/mL	Injectable	Merial	1
Melatonin	Melatonin	0.3 mg, 1.5 mg, 3 mg	Tablet, regular or extended release	Multiple	D
Meloxicam	Mobic	7.5 mg, 15 mg	Tablet	Boehringer Ingelheim	3

Generic Name	Proprietary Name	Strength	Form	Source	Approval
Meloxicam	Metacam	5 mg/mL	Injectable	Boehringer Ingelheim	1
Meloxicam	Metacam	1.5 mg/mL	Oral suspension	Boehringer Ingelheim	1
Melphalan	Alkeran	2 mg	Tablet	Celgene	3
Melphalan	Alkeran	50 mg in single use vials with 10 mL vial of sterile diluent	Powder for injection	Celgene	3
Meperidine hydrochloride	Demerol	25 mg/mL, 50 mg/mL, 75 mg/mL, 100 mg/mL	Injectable	Abbott	3
Meperidine hydrochloride	Demerol	50 mg, 100 mg	Tablet	Sanofi-Synthelabo	3
Meperidine hydrochloride	Demerol	50 mg/5 mL	Oral syrup	Sanofi-Synthelabo	3
Mephenytoin	Mesantoin	100 mg	Tablet	Novartis	3
Mepivacaine	Carbocaine	1%, 1.5%, 2%, 3%	Injectable	Multiple	3
6-Mercaptopurine	Purinethol, generic	50 mg	Tablet	GlaxoSmithKline	3
Mercaptopurine	Generic	50 mg	Tablet	Multiple	3
Meropenem	Merrem I.V.	500 mg, 1 g	Injectable	Zeneca	3
Mesalamine	Apriso	250 mg, 500 mg	Capsule, extended release	Shire	3
Mesalamine	Mesalamine	4 g/60 mL	Enema	Teva	3

Generic Name	Proprietary Name	Strength	Form	Source	Approval
Mesalamine	Canasa	1 g	Rectal suppository	Axcan Scandipharm	3
Mesna	Mesnex	100 mg/mL	Injectable	Baxter Healthcare	3
Mesna	Mesnex	400 mg	Tablet	Baxter Healthcare	3
Metaflumizone	Promaris-Cats	0.81 mL-1.6 mL	Topical	Fort Dodge	
Metaflumizone/amitraz	Promaris-Dogs	0.67 mL, 1.35 mL, 3.39 mL, 5.4 mL	Topical	Fort Dodge	
Metaproterenol sulfate	Alupent	0.65 mg/puff	Aerosol, metered	Boehringer Ingelheim	3
Metaproterenol sulfate	Alupent	0.4%, 0.6%	Solution, inhalation	Boehringer Ingelheim	3
Metaproterenol sulfate	Metaproterenol Sulfate	10 mg/5 mL	Oral syrup	Novex	3
Metaproterenol sulfate	Metaproterenol Sulfate	10 mg, 20 mg	Tablet	Teva	3
Metaraminol bitartrate	Aramine	10 mg/mL	Injectable	Merck	3
Metformin hydrochloride	Glucophage	1 g	Tablet	Bristol-Myers Squibb	3
Metformin hydrochloride	Glucophage	500 mg, 850 mg	Tablet	Bristol-Myers Squibb	3
Metformin hydrochloride	Glucophage XR	500 mg	Tablet, extended release	Bristol-Myers Squibb	3
Methazolamide	Glauc-Tabs	25 mg, 50 mg	Tablet	Akorn	3

Generic Name	Proprietary Name	Strength	Form	Source	Approval
Methenamine Hippurate	Urex	1 g	Tablet	3M	3
Methenamine mandelate	Mendelamine	0.5 g, 1 g	Tablet	Warner Chilcott	3
Methenamine mandelate	Hiprex	50 mg/mL, 100 mg/mL	Oral suspension	Aventis	3
Methicillin	Staphcillin	0.9 g, 3.6 g, 5.4 g	Injectable	Apothecon	3
Methimazole	Tapazole	5 mg, 10 mg	Tablet	Lilly	3
Methocarbamol	Robaxin V	500 mg	Tablet	Fort Dodge	1, 2
Methocarbamol	Robaxin V	100 mg/mL	Injectable	Fort Dodge	1, 2, 4
Methohexital sodium	Brevital	2.5 g/vial	Injectable	Lilly	3
Methohexital sodium	Brevital Sodium	2.5 mg/mL, 25 mg/mL	Injectable	Xanodyne	3
Methotrexate sodium	Methotrexate LPF Sodium	2.5 mg/mL, 25 mg/mL	Injectable	Abraxis	3
Methotrexate sodium	Trexal	2.5 mg, 5 mg, 7.5 mg, 10 mg, 15 mg	Tablet	Barr	3
Methoxamine hydrochloride	Vasoxyl	20 mg/mL	Injectable	GlaxcoSmithKline	3
Methoxyflurane	Metofane	99.90%	Inhalant	Abbott	3
Methscopolamine	Pamine, generic	2.5 mg, 5 mg	Tablet	Boca Pharmacal	3

Generic Name	Proprietary Name	Strength	Form	Source	Approval
Methylcellulose	Citrucel	2 g/packet	Powder for oral solution	Multiple	OTC
Methylene blue	New methylene blue, generic	10 mg/mL	Injectable	Multiple	3
Methylene blue	Urolene Blue	65 mg	Tablet	Star	3
Methylphenidate	Ritalin	5 mg, 10 mg, 20 mg	Tablet	Multiple	3
Methylphenidate	Methylphenidate	2.5 mg, 5 mg, 10 mg	Tablet, chewable	Mallinckrodt	3
Methylphenidate	Methylphenidate	20 mg, 30 mg, 40 mg	Capsule, extended release	UCB	3
Methylphenidate	Ritalin-SR	10 mg, 18 mg, 20 mg, 27 mg, 36 mg, 54 mg	Tablet, extended release	Multiple	3
Methylprednisolone	Medrol	2 mg, 4 mg, 8 mg, 16 mg, 24 mg, 32 mg	Tablet	Pfizer	3
Methylprednisolone acetate	Depo-Medrol	20 mg/mL, 40 mg/mL, 80 mg/mL	Injectable	Pharmacia and UpJohn, Boehringer Ingelheim	1, 2, 3
Methylprednisolone acetate/aspirin	Cortaba	0.5 mg/300 mg	Tablet	Pharmacia and UpJohn	1
Methylprednisolone sodium succinate	Solu-Medrol	40, 125, 500 mg/vial 1 and 2 g/vial	Injectable	Pfizer	3
4-Methylpyrazole 5% (fomepizole)	Antizol-Vet	1 g/mL	Injectable	Orphan Medical Inc	2
Methyltestosterone	Android, generic	10 mg, 25 mg	Tablet	Valeant Pharmaceuticals International, others	3
Metoclopramide	Reglan	5 mg, 10 mg	Tablet	Wyeth-Ayerst	3

Generic Name	Proprietary Name	Strength	Form	Source	Approval
Metoclopramide	Metoclopramide Intensol	1 mg/mL, 10 mg/mL	Oral solution	Roxane	3
Metoclopramide	Reglan	5 mg/mL	Injectable	Wyeth-Ayerst	3
Metoprolol	Lopressor	50 mg, 100 mg	Tablet	Novartis	3
Metoprolol	Toprol XL	25 mg, 50 mg, 100 mg, 200 mg	Tablet, extended release	AstraZeneca	3
Metoprolol	Lopressor	1 mg/mL	Injectable	Novartis	3
Metronidazole	Flagyl IV	500 mg/vial	Injectable	Pharmacia	3
Metronidazole	Flagyl, generic	250 mg, 500mg	Tablet	Pharmacia and Searle, others	3
Metronidazole	Flagyl ER	750 mg	Tablet, extended release	Pharmacia	3
Metronidazole	Flagyl	375 mg	Capsule	G.D. Searle and Company	3
Mexiletine	Mexitil	150 mg, 200 mg, 250 mg	Capsule	Multiple	3
Miconazole	Monistat-Derm	2%	Topical cream	Johnson and Johnson	3
Miconazole	Monistat 3	200 mg	Vaginal suppository	Ortho-McNeil Pharmaceuticals	3
Midazolam	Versed	1 mg/mL, 5 mg/mL	Injectable	Roche	3
Midazolam	Versed	2 mg/mL	Oral syrup	Roche	3

Generic Name	Proprietary Name	Strength	Form	Source	Approval
Mifepristone	Mifeprex	200 mg	Tablet	Danco Laboratories	3
Milbemycin oxime	Interceptor	2.3 mg, 5.75 mg, 11.5 mg, 23 mg	Tablet	Novartis	1, 2
Milbemycin oxime	Sentinel	46 mg, 115 mg, 230 mg, 460 mg (with nitenpyram)	Tablet	Novartis	1
Milrinone lactate	Primacor	1 mg base/mL	Injectable	Apotex	3
Milrinone lactate	Primacor in Dextrose 5% in plastic container	EQ 20 mg base/100 mL	Injectable	Apotex	3
Minocycline	Minocin	50 mg, 100 mg	Capsule	Lederle	3
Minocycline	Minocin	50 mg/5 mL	Oral suspension	Lederle	3
Minocycline	Minocin	100 mg/vial	Injectable	Lederle	3
Mirtazapine	Mirtazapine	15 mg, 30 mg, 45 mg	Tablet	Multiple	3
Misoprostol	Cytotec	100 μg, 200 μg	Tablet	Searle	3
Mitotane (o,p'-DDD)	Lysodren	500 mg	Tablet	Bristol-Myers Oncology	3
Mitoxantrone	Novantrone	2 mg/mL	Injectable	Serono	3
Monensin	Rumensin	20 mg/lb, 30 mg/lb, 45 mg/lb, 60 mg/lb, 80 mg/lb, 90.7 mg/lb	Premix	Elanco	4
Montelukast sodium	Singulair	Eq 10 mg base	Tablet	Merck	3

Generic Name	Proprietary Name	Strength	Form	Source	Approval
Morphine SO$_4$	Astramorph P/F	0.5 mg/mL, 1 mg/mL	Injectable	AstraZeneca	3
Morphine SO$_4$	Morphine Sulfate	10 mg, 15 mg, 30 mg	Tablet	Ranbaxy	3
Morphine SO$_4$	MS Contin	15 mg, 30 mg, 60 mg, 100 mg, 200 mg	Tablet, controlled release	Purdue-Frederick	3
Morphine SO$_4$	Avinza	20 mg, 30 mg, 50 mg, 60 mg, 90 mg, 100 mg, 120 mg	Capsule, extended release	Ligand	3
Morphine SO$_4$	Morphine Sulfate	10 mg/5 mL, 20 mg/5 mL	Oral solution	Roxane	3
Morphine SO$_4$	Morphine Sulfate	5 mg, 10 mg, 20 mg, 30 mg	Rectal suppository	Multiple	3
Moxidectin	ProHeart	30 mg, 60 mg, 136 mg	Tablet	Fort Dodge	1
Moxidectin	Cydectin	0.5% (5 mg/mL)	Pour on topical	Fort Dodge	4
Moxidectin	Quest	20 mg/mL	Oral gel	Fort Dodge	4, OTC
Moxidectin (with praziquantel)	Quest Plus	20 mg/mL (125 mg/mL praziquantel)	Oral gel	Fort Dodge	4, OTC
Mycophenolate mofetil	Cellcept	250 mg	Capsule	Roche	3
Mycophenolate mofetil	Cellcept	500 mg	Tablet	Roche	3
Mycophenolate mofetil	Cellcept	500 mg/vial	Injectable	Roche	3
Nadolol	Corzide	40 mg, 80 mg (with 5 mg bendroflumethiazide)	Tablet	King Pharmaceuticals	3

APPENDIX B: ALPHABETICAL LISTING OF DRUGS BY GENERIC AND PROPRIETARY NAME AND SOURCE

Generic Name	Proprietary Name	Strength	Form	Source	Approval
Nafcillin	Nafcillin Sodium	0.5 mg, 1 mg, 2 mg, 10 mg base/vial	Injectable	Sandoz	3
Nalbuphine	Nubain	10 mg/mL, 20 mg/mL	Injectable	Endo Pharmaceutical	3
Nalmefene hydrochloride	Revex	EQ 0.1 mg, 1 mg base/mL	Injectable	Baxter Healthcare	3
Nalorphine hydrochloride	Nalline	5 mg/mL	Injectable	Merial	1
Naloxone hydrochloride	Narcan	0.02 mg/mL, 0.4 mg/mL, 1 mg/mL	Injectable	Dupont Pharm	3
Naltrexone	Revia	50 mg	Tablet	Bristol-Myers Squibb	3
Nandrolone decanoate	Deca-Durabolin	100 mg/mL, 200 mg/mL	Injectable	Organon	3
Nandrolone phenpropionate	Durabolin	25 mg/mL, 50 mg/mL	Injectable	Organon	3
Naproxen	Naprosyn	125 mg/5 mL	Oral suspension	Roche	3
Naproxen	EC-Naprosyn	375 mg, 500 mg	Tablet, delayed release	Roche	3
Naproxen	Aleve, generic	200 mg, 250 mg, 375 mg, 500 mg	Tablet, capsule, gel caps	Bayer, others	3, OTC
Natamycin	Natacyn	5%	Ophthalmic solution	Alcon	3
Neomycin	Biosol	200 mg/mL	Oral liquid	Pharmacia	4, OTC
Neomycin	Neomix AG 325 Soluble Powder		Soluble powder	Pharmacia and UpJohn	4, OTC

Generic Name	Proprietary Name	Strength	Form	Source	Approval
Neomycin	Neomycin 325	325 g/lb	Water/feed additive	Durvet	4, OTC
Neomycin	Neo-Sol 50	71.5 g (EQ to 50 g neomycin)	Water medication	Alpharma	4, OTC
Neomycin		500 mg	Tablet	Multiple	3
Neomycin	Neo-fradin	25 mg/mL	Oral solution	Pharma-Tek	3
Neostigmine	Prostigmin	0.25 mg/mL, 0.5 mg/mL, 1 mg/mL	Injectable	ICN Pharmaceuticals	3
Nicotinamide (Vitamin B3)		Niacin	100 mg, 500 mg	Tablet	OTC 3
Nifedipine	Procardia	10 mg, 20 mg	Capsule	Pfizer	3
Nifedipine	Adalat CC	30 mg, 60 mg, 90 mg	Tablet, extended release	Bayer	3
Nifurtimox	Lampit	NI	NI	NI	5
Nikethamide	Coramine	Available in multipreparation products	NI	NI	D
Nitazoxanide	Navigator	32%	Paste	IDEXX	4
Nitenpyram	Capstar	11.4 mg, 57 mg	Tablet	Novartis	1, 2
Nitrofurantoin	Macrobid	25 mg, 50 mg, 100 mg	Capsule	Procter and Gamble	3
Nitrofurantoin	Furadantin	5 mg/mL	Oral suspension	Dura	3

Generic Name	Proprietary Name	Strength	Form	Source	Approval
Nitroglycerin	Nitro-Bid	5 mg/mL	Injectable	Aventis Pharmaceuticals	3
Nitroglycerin 2% ointment	Nitro-Bid	2%	Topical ointment	Hoeschst Marion Roussel	3
Nitroglycerin	Minitran	0.1 mg/hr, 0.2 mg/hr, 0.3 mg/hr, 0.4 mg/hr, 0.6 mg/hr, 0.8 mg/hr	Transdermal patch	3 M	3
Nitroprusside	Nitropress	50 mg/vial	Injectable	Abbott	3
Nizatidine	Axid AR	75 mg	Tablet	Whitehall-Robins	3, OTC
Nizatidine	Axid	150 mg, 300 mg	Capsule	Eli Lilly	3
Norepinephrine bitartrate	Levophed, generic	EQ 0.1 mg, 1 mg base/mL	Injectable	Multiple	3
Norfloxacin	Noroxin	400 mg	Tablet	Merck	3
Nystatin	Mycolog	OTC	Topical	Multiple	3
Nystatin	Nilstat	100,000 Units/mL	Oral suspension	Lederle	3
Nystatin	Nilstat	50 million Units, 150 million Units, 500 million Units, 1 billion Units, 2 billion Units, 5 billion Units	Bulk powder	Lederle	3
Nystatin	Mycostatin	500,000 Units	Tablet	Apothecan	3
Octreotide acetate	Sandostatin	0.05 mg/mL, 0.1 mg/mL, 0.2 mg/mL, 0.5 mg/mL, 1 mg/mL in 1 mL vials	Injectable	Novartis	3

Generic Name	Proprietary Name	Strength	Form	Source	Approval
Octreotide acetate	Generic	10 mg/5 mL, 20 mg/5 mL, 30 mg/ 5 mL in kits with 2 mL diluent	Injectable	Novartis	3
Ofloxacin	Oflaxacin	40 mg/mL	Injectable	Bedford	3
Ofloxacin	Oflaxacin	0.30%	Ophthalmic drops/solution	Bausch and Lomb	3
Ofloxacin	Floxin Otic	0.30%	Otic drops/solution	Daiici	3
Ofloxacin	Oflaxacin	200 mg, 300 mg, 400 mg	Tablet	Teva	3
Olsalazine	Dipentum	250 mg	Capsule	Celltech	3
Olsetamivir	Tamiflu	75 mg	Capsule	Hoffman La-Roche	3
Omeprazole	Prilosec, generic	10 mg, 20 mg, 40 mg	Capsule, delayed release	AstraZeneca, others	3, OTC
Omeprazole	Gastrogard	2.28 g per syringe	Oral paste	Merial	4
Omeprazole	Prilosec, generic	10 mg, 20 mg, 40 mg	Capsule	AstraZeneca, others	3, OTC
Ondansetron	Zofran	2 mg/mL, 32 mg/50 mL	Injectable	GlaxoSmithKline	3
Ondansetron	Zofran	4 mg, 8 mg, 24 mg	Tablet (and orally disentegrating)	GlaxoSmithKline	3
Ondansetron	Zofran	4 mg/5 mL	Oral solution	GlaxoSmithKline	3

Generic Name	Proprietary Name	Strength	Form	Source	Approval
Orbifloxacin	Orbax	5.7 mg, 22.7 mg, 68 mg	Tablet	Schering-Plough Animal Health	1, 2
Orgotein	Palosein	5 mg/mL	Injectable	Oxis International	1
Oxacillin	Bactocill	250 mg, 500 mg	Capsule	GlaxoSmithKline	3
Oxacillin	Bactocill	250 mg/5 mL	Oral solution	GlaxoSmithKline	3
Oxacillin	Bactocill	500 mg vials, 1 g, 2 g, 10 g vials	Injectable	GlaxoSmithKline	3
Oxazepam	Serax	10 mg, 15 mg, 30 mg	Capsule	Wyeth-Ayerst	3
Oxazepam	Serax	15 mg	Tablet	Wyeth-Ayerst	3
Oxfendazole	Synanthic	90.6 mg/mL	Oral suspension	Fort Dodge	4, OTC
Oxfendazole	Synanthic	185 mg/g	Oral paste	Fort Dodge	4, OTC
Oxtriphylline	Choledyl SA	400 mg, 600 mg	Tablet, extended release	Parke Davis/Warner Chilcott	3
Oxybutynin	Ditropan	5 mg	Tablet	Janssen	3
Oxybutynin chloride	Ditropan XL	5 mg, 10 mg, 15 mg	Tablet, extended release	ALZA	3
Oxymetholone	Anadrol-50	50 mg	Tablet	Unimed	3
Oxymetholone	Anadrol	50 mg	Tablet	Roche Laboratories	3

Generic Name	Proprietary Name	Strength	Form	Source	Approval
Oxymorphone	Numorphan	1 mg/mL, 1.5 mg/mL	Injectable	Endo Pharmaceutical	3
Oxymorphone	Numorphan	5 mg	Rectal suppository	Endo Pharmaceutical	3
Oxytetracycline	Terramycin	250 mg	Tablet	Pfizer	3
Oxytetracycline	Terramycin	50 mg/mL, 125 mg/mL	Injectable	Pfizer	3
Oxytocin	Pitocin, others	10 Units/mL	Injectable	Parke-Davis, others	3
Paclitaxel	Taxol	6 mg/mL	Injectable	Bristol-Myers Squibb	3
Pamidronate	Aredia	60 mg/vial	Injectable	Novartis	3
Pancreatic enzyme	Viokase	NA	Tablet	Axcan Pharma	3
Pancuronium bromide	Pavulon	1 mg/mL, 2 mg/mL	Injectable	Organon	3
Paromomycin (aminosidine)	Humatin	250 mg (of paromomycin)	Capsule	Monarch Pharmaceuticals	3
Paroxetine	Paxil	10 mg, 20 mg, 30 mg, 40 mg	Tablet	GlaxoSmithKline	3
Paroxetine	Paxil CR	12.5 mg, 25 mg, 37.5 mg	Tablet, controlled release	GlaxoSmithKline	3
Paroxetine	Paxil	2 mg/mL	Oral suspension	GlaxoSmithKline	3
Parvaquone	Parvaquone	EQ 5 mg base	Capsule	Novartis	3

Generic Name	Proprietary Name	Strength	Form	Source	Approval
D-Penicillamine	Depen	250 mg	Tablet	Medpointe Pharma	3
D-Penicillamine	Cuprimine	125 mg, 250 mg	Capsule	Aton Pharma	3
Penicillin G aqueous (potassium or sodium)	Pfizerpen	1 million Units, 5 million Units, 20 million Units/vial	Injectable	Pfizer	3
Penicillin G benzathine	Bicillin L-A	0.6 million Units, 1.2 million Units, 2.4 million Units/dose	Injectable IM	Monarch Pharmaceuticals	3
Penicillin G benzathine	Bicillin	300,000 Units/mL	Itramuscular suspension	Monarch Pharmaceuticals	3
Penicillin G benzathine	Bicillin	900,000 Units/2 mL, 300,000 Units/2 mL, 600,000 Units/mL	Injectable suspension	Monarch Pharmaceuticals	3
Penicillin G procaine	Penicillin G Procaine	600,000 Units/vial, 1.2 million Units/vial	Injectable	Monarch Pharmaceuticals	3
Penicillin G procaine	Crysticillin 300 A.S.	300,000 Units/mL	Injectable	Fort Dodge	4, OTC
Penicillin G procaine	Go-Dry	100,000 Units/mL	Injectable (use in dry cows only)	G.C. Hanford	4, OTC
Penicillin G, benzathine and procaine (Penicillins)	Ambi-Pen	150,000 Units/mL (Benzathine), 150,000 Units/mL (Procaine)	Injectable	Butler	4
Penicillin G, benzathine and procaine	Bicillin C-R	600,000 Units/dose (300,000 K Units each), 1.2 million Units/dose (600,000 each), 2.4 million Units/dose (1.2 million Units each)	Injectable	Monarch Pharmaceuticals	3
Penicillin G, benzathine and procaine	Bicillin C-R 900/300	1.2 million Units/dose (900,000 Units Benzathine and 300,000 Units Procaine)	Injectable	Monarch Pharmaceuticals	3

Generic Name	Proprietary Name	Strength	Form	Source	Approval
Pentamidine isethionate	Pentam	300 mg/vial	Injectable	Am Pharm Partners	3
Pentamidine isethionate	Nebupent	300 mg/vial, 600 mg/vial	Inhalation solution	Am Pharm Partners	3
Pentazocine	Talwin	30 mg/mL	Injectable	Abbott	3
Pentobarbital sodium	Pentobarbital Injection	50 mg/mL	Injectable	Wyeth-Ayerst	3
Pentobarbital sodium	Sodium Pentobarbital Injection	65 mg/mL	Injectable	Butler, J.A. Webster	1, 2
Pentobarbital sodium		100 mg	Capsule	Generic	3
Pentobarbital sodium	Nembuta	20 mg/5 mL	Elixir	Abbott	3
Pentosan polysulfate	Elmiron	100 mg	Capsule	Baker Norton	3
Pentoxifylline	Trental, generic	400 mg	Tablet, controlled/extended release	Hoechst Marion Roussel, others	3
Phenamidine isethionate	Fenamiphos	NA	NA	NA	5
Phenobarbital	Solfoton, generic	15 mg, 16 mg, 30 mg, 60 mg, 90 mg, 100 mg	Tablet	ECR Pharmaceuticals, others	3
Phenobarbital	Luminal	15 mg/5 mL, 20 mg/5 mL	Elixir		3
Phenobarbital	Luminal Sodium	30 mg/mL, 60 mg/mL, 65 mg/mL, 130 mg/mL	Injectable	Sanofi Winthrop	3
Phenoxybenzamine hydrochloride	Dibenzyline	10 mg	Capsule	Wellspring Pharmaceuticals	3

Generic Name	Proprietary Name	Strength	Form	Source	Approval
Phentolamine mesylate	Regitine	5 mg/vial	Injectable	Novartis	3
Phenylbutazone	Bizolin 100	100 mg	Tablet	Boehringer Ingelheim	1
Phenylbutazone	Phenylzone Paste	6 g, 12 g/syringe	Oral paste	Schering-Plough Animal Health	4
Phenylbutazone	Amtech Phenylbutazone 20% Injection	200 mg/mL	Injectable	Phoenix Scientific	1,4
Phenylephrine	NeoSynephrine	1% (10 mg/mL)	Injectable	Sanofi Winthrop	3
Phenylephrine	AH-chew D	10 mg	Tablet, chewable	WE Pharm	3
Phenylpropanolamine hydrochloride	Cystolamine	75 mg	Capsule, timed release	VPL	1
Phenylpropanolamine hydrochloride	Proin Drops	25 mg/mL, 50 mg/mL	Oral solution	PRN Pharmacal	1
Phenytoin	Dilantin	50 mg	Tablet, chewable	Parke Davis	3
Phenytoin	Dilantin Kapseals	30 mg, 100 mg, 200 mg, 300 mg	Capsule	Parke Davis	3
Phenytoin	Phenytoin Sodium	50 mg/mL	Injectable	Elkins-Sinn	3
Phenytoin	Dilantin-125, generic	25 mg/mL	Oral solution	Parke Davis	3
Phenytoin	Extended	30 mg, 100 mg, 200 mg, 300 mg	Capsule	Mylan	3
Phenytoin	Beuthanasia-D-Special	50 mg/mL with 390 mg/mL pentobarbital	Injectable	Schering-Plough Animal Health	1

Generic Name	Proprietary Name	Strength	Form	Source	Approval
Phosphate, potassium		3 mM phosphate and 4 mEq of sodium/mL	Injectable	Generic	3
Phosphate, sodium		3 mM phosphate and 4.4 mEq of potassium/mL	Injectable		
Physostigmine	Antilirium	1 mg/mL, 1 mg	Injectable or tablet	Forrest Pharmaceuticals	3
Physostigmine	Eserine Salicylate	0.50%	Ophthalmic solution	Alcon	3
Physostigmine	Eserine Sulfate	0.25%	Ophthalmic ointment	CIBA Vision	3
Phytomenadione (Vitamin K₁)	Aquamephyton	2 mg/mL	Injectable	Merck	3
Phytomenadione (phytonadione)	Mephyton	5 mg	Tablet	Merck	3
Phytomenadione (phytonadione)	K-Caps	25 mg	Capsule	Vetus	1, 2
Phytomenadione (phytonadione)	Vitamin K₁	10 mg/mL	Injectable	Butler	1, 2, 4
Pilocarpine hydrochloride	Pilopine HS	4%	Ophthalmic gel	Alcon	3
Pilocarpine hydrochloride	Salagen	5 mg, 7.5 mg	Tablet	MGI Pharma Inc	3
Pimobendan	Vetmedin	1.25 mg, 2 mg	Tablet	Boehringer Ingelheim	1
Pimozide	Orap	1 mg, 2 mg	Tablet	TEVA	3
Piperacillin sodium	Pipracil	2 g, 3 g, 4 g, 40 g base/vial	Injectable	AM Pharm	3

Generic Name	Proprietary Name	Strength	Form	Source	Approval
Piperacillin (with tazobactam)	Zosyn	2 g (with 250 mg), 3 g (with 375 mg), 4 g (with 500 mg), 36 g (with 4.5 g) base/vial	Injectable	Wyeth Pharms Inc	3
Piperazine	Pipa-tabs, generic	50 mg, 250 mg base	Tablet	Vet-A-Mix, others	1, 2
Piperazine citrate	Piperazine Citrate	EQ 500 mg base/5 mL	Oral syrup	Luitpold	3
Piperazine citrate	Piperazine Citrate	EQ 500 mg base/5 mL	Oral syrup	Lannett	3
Piperazine citrate	Piperazine Citrate	EQ 250 mg base	Tablet	Impax Labs	3
Pirbuterol acetate	Maxaire	EQ 0.2 mg/puff	Metered aerosol	Graceway	3
Piroxicam	Feldene, generic	10 mg, 20 mg	Capsule	Pfizer, others	3
Plicamycin	Mithracie	2.5 mg/vial	Injectable	Pfizer	3
Polyethylene glycol electrolyte solution	Miralax, generic	17 g/scoopful	Powder for recombination (for oral solution)	Braintree, others	3
Polymyxcin B	Aerosporin	500,000 Units	Injectable	Glaxosmithkline	3
Polysulfated glycosaminoglycans	Adequan I.A.	250 mg/mL	Injectable	Luitpold	1
Ponazuril	Marquis Paste	150 mg/mL	Oral paste	Bayer	4
Potassium chloride	Kaon	5 mEq	Tablet, chewable	Savage	3
Potassium chloride	Kaon	5 mEq	Tablet, coated	Adria	3

Generic Name	Proprietary Name	Strength	Form	Source	Approval
Potassium chloride	Kaon	4.68 g/15 mL	Elixir	Adria	3
Potassium chloride	Kaon	20 mEq/mL	Oral solution	Savage	3
Potassium chloride	Kaon-Cl	40 mEq/15 mL	Oral solution	Savage	3
Potassium chloride	KayCiel	20 mEq KCl in 1.5 g/packet	Powder for oral solution	Forest Pharmaceuticals	3
Potassium chloride	KayCiel	1.5 g/15 mL	Oral solution	Forest Pharmaceuticals	3
Potassium citrate	Urocit-K	5 mEq, 10 mEq extended release	Tablet	Mission Pharma	3
Potassium gluconate	Tumil-K, others	2 mEq	Tablet	Virbac	D
Potassium gluconate	Tumil-K, others	20 mEq/15 mL	Oral solution	Virbac	D
Potassium iodide	SSKI Solution	1 g/mL	Oral solution	Upsher-Smith	3
Potassium permanganate (1:2,000)	Potassium permanganate-KMnO4	NI	NI	NI	
Povidone-iodine	Betadine	5%	Ophthalmic solution	Alcon	3
Povidone-iodine	Betadine	10%	Gauze	Purdue-Frederick	3
Povidone-iodine	Betadine	0.50%	Mouthwash	Purdue-Frederick	3
Povidone-iodine	Betadine	7.50%	Shampoo	Purdue-Frederick	3

Generic Name	Proprietary Name	Strength	Form	Source	Approval
Povidone-iodine	Betadine	5%	Spray	Purdue-Frederick	3
Povidone-iodine	Betadine	10%	Swab	Purdue-Frederick	3
Povidone-iodine	Betadine	5%	Topical cream	Purdue-Frederick	3
Pralidoxime chloride	2PAM	300 mg/mL	Injectable	Meridine	3
Praziquantel	Droncit	5.86 mg/mL	Injectable	Bayer	1, 2
Praziquantel	Droncit	34 (dog), 23 (cat)	Tablet	Bayer	1, 2
Prazosin hydrochloride	Minipress	2.5 mg, 5 mg	Tablet, extended release	Pfizer	3
Prednisolone acetate	Prednisolone Acetate	25 mg/mL, 50 mg/mL	Injectable	Steris	3
Prednisolone acetate	Meticortelone Acetate	25 mg/mL	Injectable	Schering-Plough Animal Health	1, 2
Prednisolone acetate	Optisone	With neomycin	Ophthalmic ointment	Evsco Pharmaceuticals	1, 2
Prednisolone soidum phosphate	Prednis-A-Vet	20 mg/mL	Injectable	Anthony Products	1
Prenisolone sodium succinate	Solu-Delta-Cortef	10 mg/mL, 20 mg/mL, 50 mg/mL	Injectable	Pharmacia and Upjohn	1
Prednisolone	Prednisolone	1 mg, 2.5 mg, 5 mg	Tablet	Sperti	3
Prednisone	Meticorten	10-40 mg/mL	Injectable	Schering-Plough Animal Health	1, 2

Generic Name	Proprietary Name	Strength	Form	Source	Approval
Prednisone	Prednisone, generic	5 mg, 10 mg, 20 mg, 50 mg	Tablet	Chelsea Labs, others	3
Pregabalin	Lyrica	25 mg, 50 mg, 75 mg, 100 mg, 150 mg, 200 mg, 225 mg, 300 mg	Capsule	CP Pharms	3
Primaquine phosphate	Primaquine	15 mg	Tablet	Sanofi-Synthelabo	3
Primidone	Mylepsin	50 mg, 250 mg	Tablet	Fort Dodge	1
Primidone	Primidone	50 mg, 250 mg	Tablet	Fort Dodge	1
Procainamide	Pronestyl, generic	250 mg, 375 mg, 500 mg	Capusle	Apothecon, others	3
Procainamide	Pronestyl	100 mg/mL, 500 mg/mL	Injectable	Apothecon	3
Procarbazine	Matulane	50 mg	Capsule	Sigma-Tau	3
Prochlorperazine	Compazine	2.5 mg, 5 mg, 25 mg	Rectal suppository	GlaxoSmithKline/Able	3
Prochlorperazine	Compazine	1 mg/mL	Syrup	GlaxoSmithKline	3
Prochlorperazine	Compazine	5 mg, 10 mg, 25 mg	Tablet	GlaxoSmithKline	3
Prochlorperazine	Compazine	5 mg/mL	Injectable	GlaxoSmithKline	3
Promethazine hydrochloride	Phenergran	25 mg/mL, 50 mg/mL	Injectable	Wyeth-Ayerst	3

Generic Name	Proprietary Name	Strength	Form	Source	Approval
Promethazine hydrochloride	Phenergran	12.5 mg, 25 mg, 50 mg	Rectal suppository	Wyeth-Ayerst	3
Promethazine hydrochloride	Phenergran	12.5 mg, 25 mg, 50 mg, 5 mg/mL	Tablet or syrup	Wyeth-Ayerst	3
Propantheline bromide	Pro-banthine	7.5 mg, 15 mg	Tablet	Roberts Lab	3
Propiopromazine	Largon	20 mg/mL	Injectable	Wyeth-Ayerst	3
Propionibacterium acnes	Immuno-Regulin	NI	NI	NI	B
Propofol	Rapinovet	10 mg/mL	Injectable	Schering-Plough Animal Health	1, 2
Propofol	PropoFlo	10 mg/mL	Injectable	Abbott	1
Propranolol hydrochloride	Inderal LA	60 mg, 80 mg, 120 mg, 160 mg	Capsule, extended release	Wyeth-Ayerst	3
Propranolol hydrochloride	Inderal	1 mg/mL	Injectable	Wyeth-Ayerst	3
Propranolol hydrochloride	Inderal	10 mg, 20 mg, 40 mg, 60 mg, 80mg	Tablet	Wyeth-Ayerst	3
Propylthiouracil (PTU)	PTU, generic	50 mg	Tablet	Lederle, others	3
Prostaglandin F2-alpha	Lutalyse, Dinoprost	5 mg/mL	Injectable	Pharmacia and UpJohn	4
Protamine sulfate	Protamine sulfate injection	10 mg/mL	Injectable	Lilly	3
Protamine sulfate	Protamine sulfate injection	10 mg/mL	Injectable	AM Pharm Partners	3

Generic Name	Proprietary Name	Strength	Form	Source	Approval
Protamine sulfate	Protamine sulfate injection	10 mg/mL	Injectable	Elkins-Sinns	3
Protopam chloride	Protopam Chloride	1 g/vial	Injectable	Wyeth-Ayerst	3
Protriptyline	Vivactil	5 mg, 10 mg	Tablet	Merck	3
Pseudoephedrine	Sudafed, generic	30 mg, 60 mg	Tablet	Pfizer, others	OTC
Pseudoephedrine	Sudafed, generic	120 mg	Capsule	Pfizer, others	OTC
Pseudoephedrine	Sudafed, generic	6 mg/mL	Oral syrup	Pfizer, others	OTC
Psyllium	Fiberall	3.4 g fiber	Powder for oral solution	Multiple***	OTC
Psyllium	Fiberall	3.4 g	Wafer	Novartis	OTC
Psyllium	Fiberall	1, 250 mg	Tablet, chewable	Heritage Consumer	OTC
Psyllium	Metamucil	3 g fiber	Powder for oral solution	Procter and Gamble	OTC
Pyrantel pamoate	Nemex	2.27 mg/mL	Oral suspension	Pfizer	1
Pyridostigmine bromide	Mestinon	5 mg/mL	Injectable	ICN	3
Pyridostigmine bromide	Mestinon	60 mg, 180 mg extended release, 12 mg/mL	Tablet or oral solution	ICN	3

Generic Name	Proprietary Name	Strength	Form	Source	Approval
Pyrilamine maleate	Nisaval	25 mg	Tablet	Impax Labs	3
Pyrimethamine	Daraprim	25 mg	Tablet	GlaxoSmithKline	3
Pyrimethamine/ sulfadoxine	Fansidar	25 mg/500 mg	Tablet	Roche	3
Quinidine	Quinidine gluconate	80 mg/mL	Injectable	Lilly	3
Quinidine polygalacturonate	Cardioquin	275 mg	Tablet	NI	NI
Quinidine sulfate	Qunidine sulfate	100 mg, 200 mg, 300 mg	Tablet	Mutual Pharmaceuticals	3
Quinidine sulfate	Qunidine sulfate	300 mg extended release	Tablet	AH Robins	3
Ranitidine hydrochloride	Zantac	150 mg, 300 mg, 15 mg/mL	Tablet or syrup	GlaxoSmithKline	3
Ranitidine hydrochloride	Zantac	1 mg/mL, 25 mg/mL	Injectable	GlaxoSmithKline	3
Ribavirin	Virazole	6 mg vial	Inhalation	ICN	3
Riboflavin (Vitamin B_2)	Vitamin B_2	10-250 mg	Tablet		OTC
Rifampin	Rifadin	150 mg, 300 mg	Tablet	Aventis Pharmaceuticals	3
Rifampin	Rifadin	600 mg	Injectable	Aventis Pharmaceuticals	3
Rutin	Rutin	50 mg	Tablet	NA	D

Generic Name	Proprietary Name	Strength	Form	Source	Approval
Scopolamine	Donnatal	16.2 mg (multiingredient)	Capsule/tablet	AH Robins	3
Scopolamine	Donnatal	16.2 mg (multiingredient)	Oral elixir	AH Robins	3
Scopolamine	Generic	1 mg/72 hr	Transdermal patch	Novartis	3
Selamectin	Revolution	60 mg/mL, 120 mg/mL applicators	Topical solution	Pfizer	1, 2
Selegiline	Anipryl	2, 5, 10, 15, 30	Tablet	Pfizer	1
Selenious acid (sodium selenite)	Selenious acid	NI	NI	NI	D
Selenium	Selenium	NI	NI	NI	D
Selenium sulfide	Selenium sulfide	2.50%	Lotion/shampoo, topical	Alpharma, others	3
Senna	Senokot	8.6 mg	Tablet	Purdue	OTC
Sertraline hydrochloride	Zoloft	2 mg, 20 mg, 100 mg	Tablet	Pfizer	3
Sertraline hydrochloride		20 mg/mL in 60 mL	Oral concentrate	Pfizer	3
Sevelamer	Renagel	400 mg, 800 mg	Tablet	Genzyme	
Sevoflurane	Sevoflo	250 mL bottles	Inhalant	Abbott	1, 3
Sevoflurane	Ultane	250 mL bottles	Inhalant	Abbott	1

Generic Name	Proprietary Name	Strength	Form	Source	Approval
Silver nitrate solution 0.5%	Silvadene	1%	Cream, topical	King Pharmaceuticals	3
Silver sulfadiazine	Silvadene	1%	Cream, topical	King Pharmaceuticals	3
Skin So Soft	Skin So Soft by Avon	NI	NI	NI	OTC
Sodium bicarbonate	Baking Soda, others	Varies	Tablet, powder, injectable	NI	OTC
Sodium chloride	Adsorbanac	NI	NI	NI	NI
Sodium chloride	Ayr	NI	NI	NI	NI
Sodium chloride 5%	Muro 128	5 g/100 mL	Injectable	Baxter Healthcare	3
Sodium chloride 7.5%	Concentrated Sodium chloride	7.50%	Injectable	NI	NI
Sodium iodide 20% solution	Iodopen, generic	100 μg/mL	Injectable	Draximage	3
Sodium phosphate (p-32)	Phospho-Soda	0.67 mCi/mL	Solution, injection, oral	Mallinckrodt Pharmaceuticals	3
Sodium polystyrene sulfonate	Sodium polystyrene sulfonate	454 g/bottle	Oral, rectal powder	Carolina Medical, others	3
Sodium polystyrene sulfonate	NA	1 g/4 mL	Oral, rectal solution	Carolina Medical, others	3
Sodium stibogluconate antimony	Pentostam	NI	NI	NI	NI
Sodium sulfate	Glauber's salts	NI	NI	NI	NI

Generic Name	Proprietary Name	Strength	Form	Source	Approval
Sodium thiopental	Pentothal	25 mg/mL	Injectable	Fort Dodge	1, 2
Sodium thiosulfate 10%	Sodium thiosulfate	10%	Injectable	Taylor Pharmaceuticals	3
Sorbitol	Sorbitol	3 g/100 mL	Oral solution	Baxter Healthcare	3
Sotalol	Betapace	80 mg, 120 mg, 160 mg, 240 mg	Tablet	Berlex Laboratories	3
Spectinomycin	Spectinomycin	NA	Injectable, tablet	Fort Dodge	1
Spiramycin	Foromacidin, Rovamycin	NI	NI	NI	5
Spironolactone	Aldactone	25 mg, 50 mg, 100 mg	Tablet	G.D. Searle and Company, others	3
Spironolactone/hydro-chlorothiazide	Aldactazide	25 mg, 50 mg	Tablet	G.D. Searle and Company, others	3
Stanozolol	Winstrol	2 mg	Tablet, chewable	Pharmacia and Upjohn	1
Stanozolol	Winstrol	50 mg/mL	Injectable	Pharmacia and Upjohn	1
Staphage lysate	SPL-Serologic Types I and III	NI	NI	NI	
Streptokinase	Streptase	0.25×10^6, 0.75×10^6, 1.5×10^6 IU in 6 mL or 50 mini infusion bottles	Lypholized powder	Aventis Behring	3
Streptomycin, dihydro	Streptomycin, dihydro	1 g, 5 g	Injectable	Pfizer	3

Generic Name	Proprietary Name	Strength	Form	Source	Approval
Streptomycin, dihydro	Streptomycin, dihydro	500 mg/mL	Injectable	Norbrook	1
Streptozocin	Zanosar	1 g (100 mg/mL after reconstitution)	Powder for reconstitution	Gensia Sicor Pharmaceuticals	NA
Succimer	Chemet	100 mg	Capsule	Sanofi-Synthelabo	3
Succinylcholine	Anectine	20 mg/mL, 0.5 g vial, 1 g vial	Injectable	GlaxoSmithKline	3
Sucralfate	Carafate	1 g	Tablet	Aventis Pharmaceuticals	3
Sucralfate	Carafate	100 mg/mL	Syrup	Aventis Pharmaceuticals	3
Sufentanil	Sufenta	50 μg/mL	Injectable	Baxter Healthcare	3
Sulfadiazine	Sulfadiazine	500 mg	Tablet	Eon	3
Sulfadiazine/trimethoprim	Tribrissen	25 mg, 100 mg, 400 mg, 800 mg/ 5 mg, 20 mg, 80 mg, 160 mg	Tablet	Schering-Plough Animal Health	1
Sulfadiazine/trimethoprim	Tribrissen	200 mg/mL/40 mg/mL	Injectable	Schering-Plough Animal Health	1
Sulfadiazine/trimethoprim	Tribrissen	50 mg/mL/10 mg/mL	Injectable	Schering-Plough Animal Health	1
Sulfadiazine/trimethoprim	Tribrissen	25 mg, 100 mg, 400 mg, 800 mg/ 5 mg, 20 mg, 80 mg, 160 mg	Tablet	Fort Dodge	1
Sulfadimethoxine	Albon	5%	Oral suspension	Pfizer	1, 2
Sulfadimethoxine	Bactrovet	250 mg	Tablet	Schering-Plough Animal Health	1, 2

Generic Name	Proprietary Name	Strength	Form	Source	Approval
Sulfadimethoxine	Medicide-SDM	100 mg/mL	Injectable	Boerhinger Ingelheim	1
Sulfadimethozine/ ormetoprim	Primor	100 mg, 200 mg, 600 mg, 1000 mg/, 20 mg, 40 mg, 100 mg, 200 mg	Tablet	Pfizer	1
Sulfamethoxazole	Gantanol	500 mg	Tablet		
Sulfamethoxazole/ trimethoprim	Bactrim	80 mg/mL, 16 mg/mL	Injectable	Roche	3
Sulfamethoxazole/ trimethoprim	Bactrim	200 mg/5 mL, 40 mg/5 mL	Oral suspension	Roche	3
Sulfamethoxazole/ trimethoprim	Bactrim	400 mg, 800 mg/80 mg,160mg	Tablet	Roche	3
Sulfasalazine	Azulfidine	500 mg	Tablet	Pharmacia and Upjohn	3
Sulfasalazine	Azulfidine	250 mg/5 mL	Oral suspension	Pharmacia and Upjohn	3
Suprofen 1% ophthalmic solution	Profenal	1%	Ophthalmic solution	Alcon	3
Tamoxifen	Nolvadex	10 mg, 20 mg	Tablet	AstraZeneca Pharmaceuticals	3
Taurine	Taurine	250 mg, 500 mg, 1,000 mg	Capsule	Multiple	D
Teicoplanin	Investigational drug	NI	NI	NI	3
Tepoxalin	Zubrin	30 mg, 50 mg, 100 mg, 200 mg	Rapidly disintegrating tablet in blister packs	Schering-Plough	3

Generic Name	Proprietary Name	Strength	Form	Source	Approval
Terbinafine hydrochloride	Lamisil	1%	Gel	Novartis	3
Terbinafine hydrochloride	Lamisil	1%	Cream	Novartis	3
Terbinafine hydrochloride	Lamisil	1%	Topical solution	Novartis	3
Terbinafine hydrochloride	Lamisil	EQ 250 mg base	Tablet	Novartis	3
Terbutaline	Brethine	1 mg/mL, 2.5 mg, 5 mg	Injectable, tablet	Novartis	3
Terfenadine	Seldane	6 mg/mL, 60 mg	Oral solution, tablet	Hoechst Marion Roussel	5
Testosterone cypionate	Depo-Testosterone	100 mg/mL, 200 mg/mL	Injectable	Pharmacia and Upjohn	3
Testosterone ethanate	Testosterone Ethanate	200 mg/mL	Injectable	Steris	3
Testosterone propionate	Testosterone proprionate	25 mg/mL, 50 mg/mL, 100 mg/mL	Injectable	Steris	3
Testosterone, methyl	Android	10 mg, 25 mg	Tablet	ICN	3
Tetanus toxoid	Tetanus Toxoid	NI	NI	NI	B
Tetracycline hydrochloride	Achromycin	1%, 1.5%	Ophthalmic ointment	Lederle	3
Tetracycline hydrochloride	Achromycin	10 mg/mL	Ophthalmic suspension	Lederle	3
Tetracycline hydrochloride	Achromycin	3%	Topical ointment	Lederle	3

Generic Name	Proprietary Name	Strength	Form	Source	Approval
Tetracycline hydrochloride	Achromycin V, generic	250 mg, 500 mg	Capsule	Lederle, others	3
Tetracycline hydrochloride	Achromycin	250 mg/mL, 500 mg/mL	Injectable	Lederle	3
Tetracycline hydrochloride	Panmycin, generic	250 mg	Tablet	Pharmacia and Upjohn, others	1
Tetracycline hydrochloride	Panmycin	100 mg/mL	Oral suspension	Pharmacia and Upjohn	1, 2
2,3,2-tetramine	See Trientine				
Tetramisole	Anthelvet	NI	NI	NI	NA
Thenium closylate	Canopar	500 mg	Tablet	Schering-Plough Animal Health	1
Theophylline	Theophylline	4 mg/mL	Injectable	Abbott	3
Theophylline	Slo-phyllin	100 mg, 200 mg	Capsule	Aventis Pharmaceuticals	3
Theophylline	Theophylline	80 mg/15 mL	Oral suspension	Roxane	3
Theophylline sustained-release	Slo-Bid Gyrocaps	50 mg, 75 mg, 100 mg, 125 mg, 200 mg, 300 mg	Tablet extended release	Aventis Pharmaceuticals	3
Theophylline sustained-release	Theo-Dur	100 mg, 200 mg, 300 mg, 450 mg	Tablet extended release	King Pharmaceuticals	3
Thiabendazole	Tresaderm	40 mg with neomycin, dexamethasone	Topical solution	Merial	1, 2
Thiacetarsamide	Caparsolate	10 mg/mL	Injectable	Merial	1

Generic Name	Proprietary Name	Strength	Form	Source	Approval
Thiamine	Vitamin B₁	NI	NI	NI	D
Thiamylal sodium	Biotal	NA	Powder for injection	Boehringer Ingelheim	1, 2
Thiamylal sodium	Surital	NA	Powder for injection	Fort Dodge	1, 2
Thiethylperazine	Torecan	5 mg/mL, 10 mg	Injectable, rectal suppository, tablet	Novartis	3
Thioguanine	Thioguanine Tabloid	40 mg	Tablet	GlaxoSmithKline	3
Thiopental sodium	Pentothal	400 mg/g	Rectal suspension	Abbott	3
Thioridazine	Mellaril	10 mg, 25 mg, 25 mg, 50 mg, 100 mg, 200 mg	Tablet	Novartis	3
Thioridazine	Mellaril	30 mg/mL, 100 mg/mL	Oral solution	Novartis	3
Thiotepa	Thiotepa, generic	15 mg/vial, 30 mg/vial	Injectable	Teva, others	1
Thyroid Stimulating Hormone/thyrotropin	Thyrogen	1.1 mg/vial	Injectable	Genzyme	3
Ticarcillian/clavulanate	Timentin	3 g, 30 g ticarcillin/0.1 g, 1 g clavulanic acid	Injectable	SmithKline Beecham	3
Ticarcillin	Ticar	1 g, 3 g, 20 g, 30 g	Injectable	SmithKline Beecham	3
Tiletamine hydrochloride/ zolazepam	Telazol	50 mg tiletamine with 50 mg zolazepam	Injectable	AH Robins	1, 2
Tilmicosin	Micotil	300 mg/mL	Injectable	Elanco	4

Generic Name	Proprietary Name	Strength	Form	Source	Approval
Tinidazole	Tindamax	250 mg, 500 mg	Tablet	Mission Pharma	1
Tiopronin	Thiola	100 mg/mL	Tablet	Mission Pharma	3
Tobramycin	Nebcin	10 mg/mL, 40 mg/mL	Injectable	Lilly	3
Tobramycin	Tobrex	0.30%	Ophthalmic solution	Alcon	3
Tocainide	Tonocard	400 mg, 600 mg	Tablet	AstraZeneca Pharm	3
Tolazoline	Priscoline hydrochloride	25 mg/mL	Injectable	Novartis	3
Toltrazuril	Baycox	NI	NI	NI	
Toluene	Toluene	0.10%	Topical gel	Johnson and Johnson	3
Topiramate	Topomax	25 mg, 100 mg, 200 mg	Tablet	Ortho-McNeil	3
Topiramate	Topomax	15 mg, 15 mg	Sprinkle capsule	Ortho-McNeil	3
Tramadol	Ultram, others	50 mg, 100 mg, 200 mg, 300 mg	Tablet	Alpharma, others	3
Tretinoin	Retin-A	0.04, 0.1%	Topical gel	Johnson and Johnson	3
Triamcinolone	Vetalog	1.5 mg	Tablet	Fort Dodge	1, 2
Triamcinolone	Vetalog	0.10%	Cream	Fort Dodge	1, 2

Generic Name	Proprietary Name	Strength	Form	Source	Approval
Triamcinolone acetonide	Triamcinolone Acetonide	2 mg/mL, 6 mg/mL	Injectable	Boehringer Ingelheim	1, 2
Triamcinolone acetonide	Triamcinolone Acetonide	0.5 mg, 1.5 mg	Tablet	Boerhinger Ingelheim	1, 2
Triamterene	Dyrenium	50 mg, 100 mg	Tablet		
Trientine hydrochloride	Syprine	250 mg	Capsule	Aton Pharma	1
Trifluoperazine	Stelazine, others	1 mg, 2 mg, 5 mg, 10 mg	Tablet	Glaxo Smith-Kline, others	1
Triflupromazine	Vetame	10 mg, 25 mg	Tablet	Fort Dodge	1, 2
Triflupromazine	Vetame	20 mg/mL	Injectable	Fort Dodge	1, 2
Trifluridine ophthalmic solution	Viroptic	1%	Ophthalmic solution	Monarch Pharmaceuticals	3
Triiodothyronine, T_3	Cytobin	NI	NI	NI	
Trimeprazine	Temaril-P	5 mg, 3.75 g, 7.5 g sustained release with 2 mg prednisolone	Tablet	Pfizer	1
Trimethobenzamide	Tigan, generic	300 mg	Capsule	King Pharmaceuticals, others	1
Trimethobenzamide	Tigan, generic	100 mg/mL	Injectable	Hospira, others	1
Trimethoprim	Trimethoprim	100 mg, 200 mg	Tablet	Teva, others	3
Trimetrexate glucuronate	Neutrexin	EQ 25 mg base/vial, 200mg base/vial	Injectable	MedImmune Oncology	3

Generic Name	Proprietary Name	Strength	Form	Source	Approval
Tripelennamine	Recovr, generic	20 mg/mL	Injectable	Fort Dodge, others	1, 2
Trypan blue	Vision Blue	0.06%	Ophthalmic ointment	DORC	3
Tylosin	Tylan	1 mg/40 mL	Injectable	Elanco	1, 2
Tylosin tartrate	Tylan	NA	Oral liquid	Elanco	4
Tylosin with vitamins	Tylan Plus	NA	Powder for oral solution	Elanco	4
Urofollitropin	Fertinex	75 IU/ampule, 150 IU/ampule	Injectable IM	Serono	3
Urofollitropin	Fertinex	75 IU/ampule	Injectable SQ	Serono	3
Ursodiol (ursodeoxycholic acid)	Actigall	300 mg	Capsule	Novartis	3
Valproic acid (valproate)	Depakene	250 mg, 50 mg/mL	Capsule, oral syrup	Abbott	3
Vancomycin	Vancocin	1 g, 10 g	Injectable	Lilly	3
Vecuronium bromide	Norcuron	10 mg/mL, 20 mg/mL	Injectable	Steris	3
Verapamil hydrochloride	Calan	40 mg, 80 mg, 120 mg	Tablet	Searle	3
Verapamil hydrochloride	Calan	2.5 mg/mL	Injectable	Searle	3
Verapamil hydrochloride	Calan SR	120 mg, 180 mg, 240 mg sustained release	Tablet	Searle	3

Generic Name	Proprietary Name	Strength	Form	Source	Approval
Verapamil hydrochloride	Isoptin SR	120 mg, 180 mg, 240 mg	Tablet, extended release	Abbott	3
Verapamil hydrochloride	Isoptin	40 mg, 80 mg, 120 mg	Tablet	Abbott	3
Verapamil hydrochloride	Isoptin	2.5 mg/mL	Injectable	Abbott	3
Vidarabine	Vira-A	3%	Ophthalmic ointment	Parkdale	3
Vinblastine	Velban	10 mg	Injectable	Lilly	3
Vincristine sulfate	Oncovin, generic	1 mg/mL	Injectable	Faulding, others	3
Viokase	Viokase Powder	NA	Tablet	Axcan Pharma	3
Viokase	Viokase Tablets	NA	Tablet	Axcan Pharma	3
Vitamin A	Aquasol A	5,000 Units/mL, 50,000 Units/mL	Injectable	AstraZeneca	D
Vitamin A	Aquasol A	5,000 IU/0.1 mL	Oral liquid	AstraZeneca	D
Vitamin B complex	Becotin	NI	NI	NI	D
Vitamin B complex	Betalin complex	NI	NI	NI	D
Vitamin B_1 (thiamine)	Thiamine HCl	NI	NI	NI	D
Vitamin B_2 (riboflavin)	Vitamin B_2 (riboflavin)	NI	NI	NI	D

Generic Name	Proprietary Name	Strength	Form	Source	Approval
Vitamin C (ascorbic acid)	Ascorbic Acid	NI	NI	NI	D
Vitamin D_2	Calciferol	1.25 mg	Tablet	Schwarz Pharma	D
Vitamin D_3 (calcitriol)	Calcitriol	0.25 μg, 0.5 μg	Softgel	Teva	D
Vitamin E	Aquasol E	15 IU/0.3 mL	Oral liquid	AstraZeneca	D
Vitamin E	Eprolin	NI	NI	NI	D
Vitamin E	Natopherol	NI	NI	NI	D
Vitamin K_1 (phytonadione)	AquaMEPHYTON	10 mg/mL	Injectable	Merck	3
Vitamin K_1	AquaMEPHYTON	1 mg/0.5 mL	Injectable	Merck	3
Warfarin	Coumadin	1 mg, 2 mg, 2.5 mg, 3 mg, 4 mg, 5 mg, 6 mg, 7.5 mg, 10 mg	Tablet	Bristol-Myers Squibb	3
Xylazine	Rompun	20 mg/mL	Injectable	Bayer	1, 2
Yohimbine	Yobine	NI	NI	NI	
Zafirlukast	Accolate	10 mg, 20 mg	Tablet	AstraZeneca	3
Zidovudine	AZT, Retrovir, generic	10 mg/mL	Oral syrup	GlaxoSmithKline, others	3
Zidovudine	Generic	100 mg	Capsule	GlaxoSmithKline, others	3

Generic Name	Proprietary Name	Strength	Form	Source	Approval
Zidovudine	Generic	10 mg/mL	Injectable	GlaxoSmithKline, others	3
Zinc acetate	Zinc Acetate	NI	NI	NI	D
Zinc methionine	Zinpro	NI	NI	NI	D
Zinc sulfate	Vi-Zac, others	NI	NI	NI	D
Zonisamide	Zonegran	25 mg, 50 mg, 100 mg	Capsule	Eisai	3

[1]Code/Abbreviations

1 = dog
2 = cat
3 = human
4 = other animal
5 = withdrawn
B = biologic
Ci = curie
D = dietary supplement or nutraceutical (No FDA pre-approval)
EQ = equivalent to
NA = information not available
NE = not established

NI = no information could be found (Green Book, Orange Book, Micromedex)
NV = could not be verified
OTC = over-the-counter product
U = unknown

APPENDIX C

APPENDIX C: COMMON LATIN TERMS AND ABBREVIATIONS

Abbreviation	Latin	English
AD	auris dexter	right ear
ad lib.	ad libitum	as desired
AS	auris sinister	left ear
AU	auris uterque	each ear
b.i.d.	bis in die	twice a day, every 12 h
ft.	fiat	make
gtt (gtts)	guttatim	drop (drops)
h.	hora	hour
m.	misce	mix
o.d.	omnie die	once daily
OD	oculus dexter	right eye
OS	oculus sinister	left eye
OU	ocular uterque	each eye
PO	per os	orally
PRN	pro re nata	as needed
q.d.	quaque die	every day
q.i.d.	quarter in die	four times a day
q.o.d.	quaque other die	every other day
q.s.	quantum sufficit	as much as needed
sig. or S.	signa	label
sol.	solutio	solution
t.i.d.	ter in die	three times a day, every 8 h
tab.	tabella	tablet

APPENDIX D

Appendix D: Common Units and Conversion Factors
COMMON UNITS OF MEASURE

Unit	Abbreviation	Unit	Abbreviation
Concentration of Solutions		**Fluids**	
grams per deciliter	g/dL	deciliter (10^2 mL)	dL
grams per liter	g/L	liter (10^3 mL)	L
international units per liter	IU/L	microliter (10^{-6} L)	μL
micrograms per deciliter	μg/dL	milliliter (10^{-3} L)	mL
micromoles per liter	μmol/L		
microunits per milliliter	μU/mL	**Pressure**	
milliequivalents per liter	mEq/L	centimeters of water	cm H_2O
milligrams per deciliter	mg/dL	millimeters of mercury	mm Hg
millimoles per kilogram	mmol/kg		
millimoles per liter	mmol/L	**Time**	
milliosmoles per kilogram	mOsm/kg	every	q
parts per million	ppm	hour	hr
units per liter	Units/L or U/L	minute	min
		month	mo
Distance/Area		second	sec
centimeter	cm	week	wk
meter squared	m^2	year	yr
millimeter	mm		

Unit	Abbreviation
Weights	
grain (1 gr = 65 mg)	gr
gram (10^{-3} kg)	g
kilogram (10^3 g)	kg
microgram (10^{-6} g)	μg
milligram (10^{-3} g)	mg
nanogram (10^{-9} g)	ng
picogram (10^{-12} g)	pg

COMMON CONVERSIONS

Volume or Weight	Equivalent
1 dram	3.9 grams
1 drop (gt)	0.06 mL
15 drops	1 mL (1 cc)
1 fluid dram	3.7 mL
1 glass	240 mL (8 ounces)
1 grain	0.065 g or 65 mg
1 g	15.43 grains
1 kg	2.20 pounds (avoirdupois)
1 kg	2.65 pounds (Troy)
1 liter	1.06 quarts

Volume or Weight	Equivalent
1 liter	33.80 fluid ounces
1 measuring cup	240 mL (0.5 pint)
2 measuring cups	500 mL (1 pint)
1 mg	0.015 grain
1 mL	16.23 minims
1 minim	0.062 mL
1 ounce	31.1 g
1 ounce	30 mL or 28.35 g
1 pint	473.2 mL
1 quart	946.4 mL
1 tablespoon	15 mL
2 tablespoons	30 mL or 28.35 g
1 teacup	180 mL (6 ounces)
1 teaspoon	5 mL

TEMPERATURE CONVERSIONS

°Celsius to °Fahrenheit: (°C) (9/5) + 32°

°Fahrenheit to °Celsius: (°F-32°) (5/9)

PERCENTAGE CONVERSIONS

A. Percent weight in volume (w/v) expresses the number of grams of a constituent in 100 mL solution.

B. Percent weight in weight (w/w) expresses the number of grams of a constituent in 100 g dry matter.

C. Percent volume in volume (v/v) expresses the number of milliliters of a constituent in 100 mL solution.

D. To make a more dilute solution from a concentrated one, the following equation is useful: (% Desired * Volume Desired)/% Available = Volume of Concentrate Needed

APPENDIX E

lb	kg	Dog m^2	Cat m^2
1.1	0.5	0.064	0.063
2.2	1	0.101	0.100
3.3	1.5	0.132	0.131
4.4	2	0.160	0.159
5.5	2.5	0.186	0.184
6.6	3	0.210	0.208
7.7	3.5	0.233	0.231
8.8	4	0.255	0.252
9.9	4.5	0.275	0.273
11	5	0.295	0.292
12.1	5.5	0.315	0.312
13.2	6	0.333	0.330
14.3	6.5	0.352	0.348
15.4	7	0.370	0.366
16.5	7.5	0.387	0.383
17.6	8	0.404	0.400
18.7	8.5	0.421	0.416
19.8	9	0.437	0.433
20.9	9.5	0.453	0.449
22	10	0.469	0.464

lb	kg	Dog m²	Cat m²
23.1	10.5	0.484	0.480
24.2	11	0.500	0.495
25.3	11.5	0.515	0.509
26.4	12	0.529	0.524
27.5	12.5	0.544	0.539
28.6	13	0.558	
29.7	13.5	0.573	
30.8	14	0.587	
31.9	14.5	0.601	
33	15	0.614	
34.1	15.5	0.628	
35.2	16	0.641	
36.3	16.5	0.655	
37.4	17	0.668	
38.5	17.5	0.681	
39.6	18	0.694	
40.7	18.5	0.706	
41.8	19	0.719	
42.9	19.5	0.732	
44	20	0.744	
45.1	20.5	0.757	
46.2	21	0.769	

lb	kg	Dog m^2
47.3	21.5	0.781
48.4	22	0.793
49.5	22.5	0.805
50.6	23	0.817
51.7	23.5	0.829
52.8	24	0.840
53.9	24.5	0.852
55	25	0.864
56.1	25.5	0.875
57.2	26	0.887
58.3	26.5	0.898
59.4	27	0.909
60.5	27.5	0.920
61.6	28	0.931
62.7	28.5	0.942
63.8	29	0.953
64.9	29.5	0.964
66	30	0.975
67.1	30.5	0.986
68.2	31	0.997
69.3	31.5	1.007

APPENDIX E: CONVERSIONS OF WEIGHT TO BODY SURFACE AREA (IN SQUARE METERS) FOR DOGS AND CATS[1]

lb	kg	Dog m^2
70.4	32	1.018
71.5	32.5	1.029
72.6	33	1.039
73.7	33.5	1.050
74.8	34	1.060
75.9	34.5	1.070
77	35	1.081
78.1	35.5	1.091
79.2	36	1.101
80.3	36.5	1.111
81.4	37	1.121
82.5	37.5	1.132
83.6	38	1.142
84.7	38.5	1.152
85.8	39	1.162
86.9	39.5	1.171
88	40	1.181
89.1	40.5	1.191
90.2	41	1.201
91.3	41.5	1.211
92.4	42	1.220
93.5	42.5	1.230

lb	kg	Dog m²
94.6	43	1.240
95.7	43.5	1.249
96.8	44	1.259
97.9	44.5	1.268
99	45	1.278
100.1	45.5	1.287
101.2	46	1.297
102.3	46.5	1.306
103.4	47	1.315
104.5	47.5	1.325
105.6	48	1.334
106.7	48.5	1.343
107.8	49	1.352
108.9	49.5	1.362
110	50	1.371
111.1	50.5	1.380
112.2	51	1.389
113.3	51.5	1.398
114.4	52	1.407
115.5	52.5	1.416
116.6	53	1.425
117.7	53.5	1.434

APPENDIX E: CONVERSIONS OF WEIGHT TO BODY SURFACE AREA (IN SQUARE METERS) FOR DOGS AND CATS[1]

lb	kg	Dog m^2
118.8	54	1.443
119.9	54.5	1.452
121	55	1.461
122.1	55.5	1.470
123.2	56	1.478
124.3	56.5	1.487
125.4	57	1.496
126.5	57.5	1.505
127.6	58	1.513
128.7	58.5	1.522
129.8	59	1.531
130.9	59.5	1.539
132	60	1.548
133.1	60.5	1.557
134.2	61	1.565
135.3	61.5	1.574
136.4	62	1.582
137.5	62.5	1.591
138.6	63	1.599
139.7	63.5	1.608
140.8	64	1.616
141.9	64.5	1.624

lb	kg	Dog m^2
143	65	1.633
144.1	65.5	1.641
145.2	66	1.649
146.3	66.5	1.658
147.4	67	1.666
148.5	67.5	1.674
149.6	68	1.683
150.7	68.5	1.691
151.8	69	1.699
152.9	69.5	1.707
154	70	1.715

. . . .

Notes

[1]A formula for a more precise calculation of BSA:

$$\text{BSA in m}^2 = (K \times W^{2/3})/10^4$$

Given that: BSA = body surface area

m^2 = square meters

W = weight in grams

K = 10.1 (dogs), 10.0 (cats)

[1]Ettinger, SJ, Feldman, EC, eds. *Textbook of Veterinary Internal Medicine*. 2nd ed. Philadelphia: Saunders; 1975.

APPENDIX F: THERAPEUTIC DRUG MONITORING DATA FOR DRUGS MONITORED IN SMALL ANIMALS

Drug Name	Therapeutic Range**	Elimination half-life	Time to steady-state[1]	Sample Collection Time: Peak	Sample Collection Time: Trough
Amikacin	2-25 μg/mL[2]	1-2 h	NR	0.75-1 h (plastic only)	2 half-lives (3-6 h)[2]
Aspirin	50-100 μg/mL	8 h (D)	NR	2-4 h	
		38 h (C)	8 days		BND
Benzodiazepines	100-200 ng/mL[3]	<8 h	NR		BND[3]
Bromide (sodium or potassium)	1-3.5 mg/mL	14-21 days	2-3 months[4]		BND
Cyclosporine	Immunosuppression: 2 h Peak: 800-1400 ng/mL	3-8[5]	NR[5]	2 h	BND (12 h)[5]
	Immunosuppression: 12 h Trough: 400-600 ng/mL				
	Inflammatory Bowel Disease: 12 h Trough 250 ng/mL				
	Perianal Fistula: 12 h Trough 100-300 ng/mL				
Digoxin	0.8-2 ng/mL	36 h	7 days	Toxicity: 2[6] (glass only)	Efficacy: BND[6] (glass only)
Gentamicin	0.5-1.5 μg/mL[2] 5-8 μg/mL	0.9-1.3 h	NR	0.75-1 h (plastic only)	2 half-lives (3-6 h)[2]
Levetiracetam	5.5-20 ng/mL	2-3.6	NR	2 h	BND
Phenobarbital	14-45 μg/mL	32-75 h	14-16 days	4-5 h[7]	BND
Primidone	Based on phenobarbital[8]	32-75 h	14-16 days	4-5 h[7]	BND

Drug Name	Therapeutic Range**	Elimination half-life	Time to steady-state 1	Sample Collection Time: Peak	Sample Collection Time: Trough
Procainamide	25-50 μg/mL[9]	2.9 h	NR	2-4 h	BND
Theophylline	10-20 μg/mL	5.7 h	NR	2 h	BND
		7.9 h	40 h	2 h	BND
Thyroxine (T4)	1-3.5 μg/dL (12.9-45 nmol/L) (D)	12-15 h (D)	NR[10]	4-6 h	BND
	1-4 μg/dL (12.9-51.5 nmol/L) (C)				
Free Thyroxine (fT4)	1-3.5 ng/dL (12.9-45 pmol/L) (D)	5-6 h (D)	NR[10]	4-6 h	BND
	1-4 ng/dL (12.9-51.5 pmol/L) (C)				
Thyronine (T3)	0.5-1.8 ng/ml (D)	5.6 h	NR		
	0.4-1.6 ng/ml (C)				
Zonisamide	10-40 μg/ml	16-65	3-10 days	2 h (D)	BND

Abbreviations

BND = before next dose

C = cat

D = dog

NR = not relevant

**Therapeutic ranges are generally extrapolated from human patients. An exception exists for antimicrobials and phenobarbital or bromide. Therapeutic ranges may also vary with the laboratory performing the assay and specifically with the instrumentation used to assay the drug of interest. Values in this table may be superseded if the values for the instrument have been validated appropriately. Because sample sizes and assay methodologies vary, the specific laboratory that will be performing the assay should be contacted regarding sample volume, proper collection tubes, need for refrigeration, and other sample handling specifics as well as "normal" ranges.

Notes

[1] Half-life = (0.693)/[Ln(peak/trough)/(trough time-peak time)]. Steady-state is generally reached in three to five elimination half-lives. Steady-state generally is not relevant (NR) for drugs whose half-life is shorter than the dosing interval. Monitoring for such drugs can occur either with the first dose or within the first day.

[2] Target peak concentrations for aminoglycosides depend on the infecting organism and its minimum inhibitory concentration (MIC). The target peak concentration should be four to 10 times the MIC. Trough concentration should be ≤ 1-2 μg/mL in order to minimize toxicity. If both efficacy and safety are the intent of monitoring, a second sample should be taken at a time when concentrations will remain detectable (i.e., one to two half-lives after the first dose).

[3] Concentrations reflect both parent compound and metabolite.

[4] If a loading dose was given, collect a single sample the day after loading (to determine what was achieved with the loading dose), three weeks later (to make sure the maintenance dose is appropriate), and again at three months from the first dose (to establish a new baseline at steady-state). If only a maintenance dose is given (i.e., no loading dose administered), collect samples at three weeks and three months.

[5] Most assays require whole blood. Ranges for immunosuppression are based on human data and the fluorescent polarized immunoassay. Trough concentrations (based on humans) achieved via high performance liquid chromatography (HPLC) are 100-300 ng/ml and concentrations achieved via radioimmunoassay (monoclonal) are 150-400 ng/ml. The laboratory performing the monitoring should be contacted to confirm therapeutic range based on their assay as well as the sample type. The cyclosporine half-life can be markedly longer in the presence of drugs which compete with it for p-glycoprotein or drug metabolizing enzymes. For atopy, trough concentrations are not likely to be detectable with dosing intervals that approach or exceed 24 hours. A peak sample might be collected. A therapeutic range has not been established for atopy; the peak target for the patient should be established once response has occurred.

[6] Elimination half-life can markedly vary with state of disease and response to drug therapy. Both peak and trough levels are recommended so that the half-life can be calculated. Because stress of sample collection may slow absorption, animals ideally should be dosed at home before collection of peak sample. Concentrations necessary for negative chronotropy may be lower than that necessary for positive inotropy.

[7] Fasting prior to collection of peak sample is recommended.

[8]Primidone is metabolized to phenobarbital. Doses are designed for phenobarbital to reach its therapeutic range. Phenobarbital is 30 times more potent than primidone as an anticonvulsant.

[9]As suggested in Papich MG, Davis LE, Davis CA. Procainamide in the dog: antiarrhythmic plasma contractions after intravenous administration. J Vet Pharmacol Therap. 1986:9;359-369. Procainamide is metabolized to an acetylated metabolite which contributes markedly to efficacy. Deficient acetylation in dogs requires higher concentrations of procainamide in dogs. Monitoring should include both the parent compound and metabolite.

[10]Values for ranges of thyroid hormones reflect the radioimmunoassay used. Values are likely to be different for each laboratory. Contact your laboratory, or if performing assays in-house, establish your own normal ranges. The overlap between normal and abnormal can be great regardless of the laboratory and interpretation should be based on clinical signs. Monitoring should not take place until the body has had a chance to physiologically adapt to drug therapy (i.e., four weeks after therapy is implemented).

APPENDIX G: EFFECTS OF DRUGS AND OTHER ARTIFACTS ON THERAPEUTIC DRUG MONITORING RESULTS

Drug	Artifact	Sequelae
All drugs	Serum separator tubes	Silicon gel can bind drug, decreasing concentrations
Aminoglycosides	Glass tubes	Glass binds drug, decreasing concentrations
	Beta-lactams	High concentrations of beta-lactam antibiotics inactivate aminoglycoside, decreasing concentrations
Bromide	Increased serum chloride	Depending on the assay, chloride cannot be distinguished from bromide, resulting in artificially high chloride concentrations
Digitalis glycosides	Rubber stoppers	Stopper may bind drug, decreasing concentrations
Phenobarbital, phenytoin, primidone	Drugs	Concentrations are decreased by phenobarbital-induced drug metabolism and other drugs that stimulate drug metabolism. Concentrations are increased by cimetidine, chloramphenicol, and other inhibitors of drug metabolism. Concentrations are increased by very high concentrations of clorazepate
Thyroid hormones	Drugs	Phenobarbital increases peripheral metabolism and may decrease concentrations
Theophylline	Drugs	Concentrations are increased by drugs that decrease metabolism, including enrofloxacin, imidazole, antifungals, cimetidine, and others

APPENDIX H: CONSTANT IV INFUSION RATES[1,2]

Drug	Indications	Loading Dose	Maintenance	Diluent
Atracurium besylate	Competitive neuromuscular blockade	0.3-0.5 mg/kg	3.6-9 μg/kg/min	5% dextrose, 0.9% NaC[l3]
Butorphanol	Mixed agonist/antagonist opioid analgesic	0.2-0.4 mg/kg	0.1-0.4 mg/kg/h	Any IV fluid
Calcium gluconate	Hypocalcemia, life-threatening hyperkalemia	None	10 mg/kg/h	Any IV fluid.[3,4] Monitor electrocardiogram
Cimetidine	Antisecretory, antiemetic	2.5 mg/kg	0.5 mg/kg/h	Any IV fluid
Cisplatin	Anticancer	None	60-70 mg/m^2 over 6 h	0.9% NaC[l3]
Dextran 70	Plasma volume expander	None	1 mL/kg/h	5% dextrose, 0.9% NaCl
Diazepam	Anticonvulsant	5-10 mg, to effect	0.2-1mg/kg/h, to effect	5% dextrose, 0.9% NaCl[3,5-7]
Diltiazem	Negative chronotrope, negative inotrope	0.15-0.25 mg/kg slow IV	5-20 μg/kg/min, to effect	Any IV fluid
Dobutamine	Positive chronotrope, positive inotrope	None	2.5-10 μg/kg/min (D) 1-5 μg/kg/min (C)	Any IV fluid[3,8] Any IV fluid[3,8]
Dopamine hydrochloride	Positive chronotrope, positive inotrope	None	5-20 μg/kg/min, to effect	Any nonalkaline IV fluid[3,9]
	Low dose (renal vasodilation)	None	1-4 μg/kg/min	Any nonalkaline IV fluid[3,9]
	Mid dose	None	5-10 μg/kg/min	Any nonalkaline IV fluid[3,9]
	High dose	None	10-20 μg/kg/min	Any nonalkaline IV fluid[3,9]

Drug	Indications	Loading Dose	Maintenance	Diluent
Epinephrine	Positive inotrope, positive chronotrope, bronchodilation (status asthmaticus)	None	0.005-1.5 μg/kg/min, to effect	Any IV fluid[7]
Esmolol	Selective beta-1 blocker: Negative chronotrope, negative inotrope (hypertension, supraventricular tachycardia)		50-200 μg/kg/min	5% dextrose, 0.9% NaCl[3,4]
Ethanol	Ethylene glycol toxicity	0.6 g/kg	100 mg/kg/h	Dilute in 0.9% NaCl to a 7% solution (7 mL ethanol in 93 mL NaCl)
Fentanyl citrate	Mu receptor opioid analgesic	None	0.7 μg/kg/h	5% dextrose[3]
		4-10 μg/kg	2-10 μg/kg/h	
	Anesthesia		50-100 μg/kg/h	
			20-100 μg/kg/h (0.33-1.66 μg/kg/min) (D)	
			10-50 μg/kg/h (0.15-0.8 μg/kg/min) (C)	
Furosemide	High ceiling loop diuretic, hypercalcemia	None	0.1-1 mg/kg/h, to effect	Any IV fluid[7]
Glucagon	For transient control of hypoglycemia	50 mg/kg	5-15 ng/kg. Maximum of 40 ng/kg	
Heparin	Disseminated intravascular coagulopathy	10-100 Untis/kg[10]	5-10 Units/kg/h[10]	Any IV fluid[3]
	Thromboembolic disease	100-300 Units/kg	10-50 Units/kg/h	

Drug	Indications	Loading Dose	Maintenance	Diluent
Hetastarch (hydroxylethyl starch)	Plasma volume expander	None	1 mL/kg/h	
Hydrocortisone sodium phosphate	Hypoadrenocorticism	1 mg/kg	0.625 mg/kg/h (D)	Any IV fluid. Dilute to 0.1-1 mg/mL
Hydromorphone	Analgesia	0.05 mg/kg	0.01-0.05 mg/kg/h	
Inamrinone	Low-output heart failure	1-3 mg/kg	30-100 μg/kg	
Insulin, regular	Hyperglycemia (ketoacidosis)		0.04-07 Units/kg/h (D)	If glucose <250 mg/dL, 0.45% NaCl + 5% D5W. If glucose > 250 mg/dL, 0.9% NaCl[2,6]
			0.034 Units/kg/h (C)	If glucose <250 mg/dL, 0.45% NaCl + 5% D5W. If glucose >250 mg/dL, 0.9% NaCl[2,6]
Isoproterenol hydrochloride	Positive chronotrope, positive inotrope	None	0.04-0.08 μg/kg/min	Any IV fluid. Dilute 1 mg in 500 mL[3]
Ketamine hydrochloride	Analgesia, with lidocaine and morphine	1 mg/kg	10 μg/kg/min (D)	
	Analgesia, subanesthetic	0.25-0.5 mg/kg	0.12-1.2 mg/kg/h	
Lidocaine	Ventricular arrhythmias	1-4 mg/kg (D)	30-80 μg/kg/min (D)	5% dextrose. 0.9% NaCl less preferred[3]
	Analgesia, with ketamine and morphine	0.25-1 mg/kg (C)	10-40 μg/kg/min	
		None	10-50 μg/mkg/min (D)	

APPENDIX H: CONSTANT IV INFUSION RATES[1,2]

Magnesium sulfate 25%	Hypomagnesemia	None	Up to 1 mEq/kg/day	5% dextrose, diluted to <20%[3]
Drug	**Indications**	**Loading Dose**	**Maintenance**	**Diluent**
Mannitol 20%	Osmotic diuretic	None	0.5-1 g/kg/h for 2-6 h	5% dextrose to a 8-10% solution[3]
		0.5 g/kg over 20-30 min	1-2 mg/kg/min	5% dextrose to a 8-10% solution[3]
	Increased intracranial or intraocular pressure	None	0.225 mg/kg for 6 h (monitor osmolarity)	5% dextrose to a 8-10% solution[3]
Medetomidine hydro-chloride	Analgesia	1 μg/kg	1-3 μg/kg/h	
	Combination analgesia	1-6 μg/kg	1-6 μg/kg/h	
Methylprednisolone sodium succinate	Spinal cord trauma	30 mg/kg	2.5 mg/kg/h for 42 hours, reducing dose gradually	5% dextrose or 0.9% NaCl[3]
Metoclopramide	Antiemetic, gastric stasis	None	0.01-0.02 mg/kg/h (D) 0.01-0.05 mg/kg/h (C)	Any IV fluid without calcium[3]
Midazolam	Anesthetic adjuvant	0.2-0.4 mg/kg IV or IM	0.2-0.5 mg/kg/h	
Milrinone		30-300 μg/kg	1-10 μg/kg/min	
Morphine SO4	Pure opioid analgesic	0.2-0.5 mg/kg (IM)	0.1-0.3 mg/kg/h (C)	5% dextrose diluted to 0.1-1 mg/mL[3]
	Analgesia with lidocaine, ketamine	None	0.12-1.2 mg/kg/h (D) 3.3 μg/kg/min (D)	
Nicardipine	Hypertension	None	0.5-5 μg/kg/min	

Drug	Indications	Loading Dose	Maintenance	Diluent
Nitroprusside	Hypertensive crisis Pulmonary edema	None None	1-10 μg/kg/min 0.5-5 μg/kg/min. Start low and increase slowly. Monitor blood pressure	5% dextrose[7,11]
Norepinephrine bitartrate	Vasopressor	None	0.05-0.2 μg/kg/min	5% dextrose[3]
Ondansetron	Antiemetic	0.5 mg/kg	0.5 mg/kg/h (0.0083 μg/kg/min)	
Oxytocin	Dystocia	None	5-10 Units over 30 min (D)	5% dextrose or 0.9% NaCl
		None	2-5 Units over 30 min (C)	
Pancuronium bromide	Neuromuscular blockade	0.04-0.1 mg/kg	0.06-0.1 mg/kg/h	5% dextrose or 0.9% NaCl
Pentobarbital	Anticonvulsant, chemical restraint	3-15 mg/kg, to effect	0.2-1 mg/kg/h	5% dextrose of 0.9% NaCl[3]
Phentolamine	Hypertension	0.05-0.1 μg/kg/min	5-30 μg/kg/min	
Phenylephrine	Vasopressor	None	1-3 μg/kg/min	5% dextrose or 0.9% NaCl
Phosphate, parenteral	Hypophosphatemia		0.01-0.18 mM/kg/h	Discontinue when serum phosphorus >2 mg/dL
Potassium chloride	Hypokalemia	None	Not to exceed 0.5 mEq/kg/h	Any IV fluid, 28-80 mEq/L

APPENDIX H: CONSTANT IV INFUSION RATES[1,2]

Drug	Indications	Loading Dose	Maintenance	Diluent
Potassium phosphate	Hypophosphatemia	None	0.01-0.03 mM/kg/h for 6 h	0.9% NaCl
Procainamide	Ventricular arrhythmias	6-8 mg/kg over 5 min (D)	25-50 μg/kg/min	0.9% NaCl
Propofol	Anesthesia	2-6 mg/kg	0.05-0.4 mg/kg/min	
Pyridostigmine	Myasthenia gravis		0.01-0.03 mg/kg/h	
Selenium				
Sodium bicarbonate	Alkalosis	None	50% of calculated dose (based on deficit) over 4-6 h	5% dextrose or 0.9% NaCl[3]
Streptokinase	Thromboembolic disease	15,000-18,000 IU/Kg	45,000 IU/h	
Streptozocin	Insulinoma		500 mg/m^2 in 18-20 mL/kg saline diuresis	In saline. Add drug during the fourth or fifth h of a 7-8 h diuresis
Sufentanil	Analgesia	1-2 μg/kg/min	0.1 μg/kg/min	
Ticarcillin (with or without clavulanate)	Susceptible infections	15-25 mg/kg	7.5-15 mg/kg/h	
Vasopressin	Vasooplegia		1-4 mUnits/kg/min	
Verapamil hydrochloride	Supraventricular arrhythmias	0.05-0.15 mg/kg	2-10 μg/kg/min	
Vitamin B complex	Thiamine deficiency, long-term IV fluid therapy	None	2-4 mL/L at maintenance fluid rate	

[1] Boothe DM. Small Animal Clinical Pharmacology and Therapeutics. Philadelphia, Pa: WB Saunders Co.; 2001.

[2] Administration of an IV drug is inherently associated with greater risk of adverse events. Become familiar with the contraindications and risks of drug administration. In general, diluted solutions should be used within 24 hours. To calculate the rate of fluid administration to a patient:
a. Dose infused (mg/kg/h): drug dose = (mg/kg) * (h) * body weight (kg) * time of infusion (h).
b. Calculate total amount of fluids to be administered during the time of infusion: fluid dose (mL/kg/hr) = dose (mL/kg) * body weight (kg) * time of infusion (h).
c. Add the calculated amount of drug to the calculated amount of fluid. To adjust to a convenient volume (e.g., 500 mL of fluid), multiply the calculated dose proportionately: drug dose (mg)/fluid dose (mL) = X/500 mL + B where X is the mg to be calculated and B is the volume to be added to 500 mL of fluid. An equivalent amount of fluid should be withdrawn or emptied from the bag prior to addition of the drug.
d. The prepared solution should be administered at the rate decided in b.

EXAMPLE: To prepare a 5 h infusion of dobutamine for a 25 kg dog:
Total dose of drug needed for the 5 h period (low to mid range of dose provided in Appendix H) = (5 μg/kg/min) * (60 min/h) * (5 h) * 25 kg = 37,500 μg = 37.5 mg.
Total dose of fluid during the 5 h period (based on approximately a 25-30 mL/kg/day of maintenance fluids) = (1 mL/kg/h) * (25 kg) * (5 h) = 125 mL.
Thus, 37.5 mg of dobutamine should be added to a total volume of 125 mL of fluid for the 5 h infusion period.
To adjust the total amount of drug added in 125 mL to a total volume of 500 mL of fluid, where X is the new total amount of drug = (X mg dobutamine)/(500 mL of fluid) = (37.5 mg dobutamine)/(125 mL) = 150 mg dobutamine.
If dobutamine is purchased as a solution prepared as 12.5 mg dobutamine/mL (Appendix B), the total volume of the dobutamine preparation needed for the 5 h infusion (and to be added to the total volume of 500 mL) = 150 mg dobutamine/(12.5 mg dobutamine/mL) = 12 mL of dobutamine.
Since the calculations are based on a total volume of 500 mL, 12 ml of fluids should be removed from the 500 mL bag of fluid prior to adding the calculated volume of 12.5 mg/mL dobutamine.

[3] Potential drug incompatibilities should preclude mixing this drug with other drugs.

[4] Due to drug incompatibilities, do not combine with sodium bicarbonate.

APPENDIX H: CONSTANT IV INFUSION RATES[1,2]

[5] Do not use if solution becomes cloudy.

[6] Drug will bind to polyvinyl plastic of IV lines. Flush fluid lines with approximately 50 mL of prepared solution prior to use/administration and use short infusion lines.

[7] Protect solution from light.

[8] Slight pink discoloration is expected.

[9] Extravasation may cause necrosis and sloughing. Treat extravasated area with 5 * 10 mg phentolamine prepared in 10-15 mL of 0.9% NaCl.

[10] Use lower dose in cats. Adjust dose based on activated partial thromboplastin time (APTT) (1.5-2.5 fold increase). Loading dose can be administered IV or, for disseminated intravascular coagulation, loading dose can be administered in an appropriate blood replacement product following a 30-minute incubation.

[11] Use drug with extreme caution. Use with infusion pump only. Death due to cyanide toxicity may occur.

LIST OF ABBREVIATIONS

Abbreviations that are used in the formulary include the following:

ACTH = adrenocorticotropin releasing hormone
AV = atrioventricular
C = cat
Ci = curie
CNS = central nervous system
D = dog
D/W = dextrose in water
EDTA = ethylenediaminetetraacetic acid
EQ = equivalent to
H = hour
IA = intraarticular
IM = intramuscular
IN = intranasal
IP = intraperitoneal

IT = intratracheal
IU = international units
IV = intravenous
MAC = mean alveolar concentration
Min = minutes
NA = not available
NE = not established
NI = not identifiable
PO = per os (by mouth)
PRN = as needed
q = every
SA = sinoatrial
SC = subcutaneous
Tbsp = tablespoon
Tsp = teaspoon

* A reminder that antimicrobial dosing regimens should be adjusted for the individual patient and that empirical selection may be limited by emerging resistance

++ Glucocorticoids generally are dosed to remission then tapered to a minimum effective dose for maintenance. Doses should be tapered as drugs are discontinued. Prednisolone is generally preferred to prednisone in cats